Overcom Amenorrhea: Get Your Period Back. Get Your Life Back.

Tina Muir

Overcoming Amenorrhea by Tina Muir

Published by Tina Muir Publish

P.O Box 54231, Lexington, KY 40509

© 2019 Tina Muir

Cover by Kevin Fox
Cover image from
www.thanksgivingdayrace.com

CONTENTS

Introduction   **8**

On Becoming the Face of Amenorrhea in the Running Community   **11**
   My Story   15

What are the Causes of Amenorrhea?   **70**
   Restricted Eating   71
   Weight and Weight Loss   75
   Exercise   77
   Exercise and Amenorrhea   78
   Control of the Menstrual Cycle   80
   Exercise and Stress   80
   Stress and the Menstrual Cycle   82
   Stress   85
   Genetics   87

Is Amenorrhea Serious? Can Amenorrhea Lead to Infertility?   **88**

What Else Could Amenorrhea Impact if Left Untreated?   **91**

Help Me Get My Period Back   **94**
   Background Check   95
   Blood Work and Further Tests   99
   Medication   101
   Seeing a Naturopath   104
   Change the Quality of Your Diet   105
   Take a Few Weeks Off   108
   Cutting Back on Training   110

Increasing Caloric Intake   118

Just a Little Extra   129

If You Think You Might Have an Eating Disorder   132

Do I REALLY Have to Stop Running?   **134**

Do I REALLY Have to Gain Weight?   **140**

Ready to Take the Plunge and Stop Running?   **150**

Find Penny   150

Journaling   152

Joy List   153

The Ultimate Bucket List   154

Gratitude List   155

If Becoming Pregnant is the Goal   157

If Health is the Goal   160

Other Recovery Secrets   **164**

Minimize Exercise   164

Remove Stress and Pressure   167

Acupuncture   169

Yoga and Meditation   171

List of Joy   172

Go Eat "Bad" Foods   176

Go Shopping   180

Other Support   **186**

YES! I Have My Period Back!   **192**

My Final Words to You, My Friend   199

Hi, friend!   **202**

Resources   **203**

Podcasts Mentioned   **204**

    Books Mentioned   205

    Other Suggested Services   205

    Other Reading Materials   206

    About the Author   207

Introduction

I had always wanted to be a mother.

Ever since I was a little girl, I knew that one day, having children of my own would be the most important thing I would ever do. I looked after my sister as if I was her mother (yes, she hated it most of the time!), and I loved being there for her. I looked forward to the day I could teach a child of my own everything I knew about the world. Helping them to grow into the best person they could be, doing their part to make the world a better place.

For some reason, I always saw a girl. Maybe because I did have a younger sister, maybe because my mum was the epitome of a caring mother and I wanted to be just like her, maybe just because every young girl loves to look after her baby girl, or maybe I just sensed that some day that would happen for me.

I envisioned us going on girls' trips together, singing to Disney songs in the car, and watching her hold hands with her daddy.

Like clouds in the sky, those thoughts would come and go as I moved on with my day, something much more pressing taking over, and I would put that memory back into storage.

Someday.

I went on to make silly mistakes as a teenager and did what I could to live my best life, as I became an adult.

It's funny, you spend most of your life trying NOT to get pregnant, desperate not to become a parent to someone else while you are still trying to figure out who YOU are, embracing your independence. And then suddenly, something changes. Deep down we all know that there is never really a "good time" to start a family, we will always have "just one more thing I want to achieve," but we know we will want to have children of our own, regardless of the timing.

Around the time starting a family was beginning to creep into my mind, knowing the day I would be ready was drawing ever closer, I started to accept that something I had been ignoring was really starting to worry me.

It had been a long time since I had a period; so long, I couldn't even tell you what year it was. I had stopped carrying tampons in my bag years before. I had forgotten the feeling of cramps. I had never worried about my racing being off because it was my "time of the month."

I was too busy making the most of the "good side" of amenorrhea. Never having to worry about it, at all.

Until it started to change the way I looked at myself, and who I wanted to be. I knew it was time to actually do something about it. I began the emotional rollercoaster that was going to force me to confront who I really was, challenge every fiber of my being in a way I never expected, and ultimately, lead to the most beautiful little girl being born less than a year after I decided I wanted that "someday" to be now.

I hope for you, this book can be a source of hope, a friend in your pocket for those tough moments to show that the other side IS worth it and a reminder that you are more than the way you look, so much more.

On Becoming the Face of Amenorrhea in the Running Community

When I admitted to the world my struggle with amenorrhea, I had no idea it would have the impact it did on the running world. I didn't expect to become the "amenorrhea girl" in all areas of sports or open up the conversation the way I did.

In a matter of a week, my story about stopping running and going through nine years of no period spread like wildfire, thanks to ESPN, *Runners World*, *Glamour*, *SELF* and many other news sources. I even had *People* magazine do a three-part feature on me, with a cool video on my story.

That is, I think, when you can say your story went viral ;)

At the time, I was thrilled to see this becoming a point of conversation. Not as thrilled to know that many women were also experiencing this, and likely the, *"What the F is wrong with my body"* feelings I had, but I took comfort knowing that by sharing my story, it was helping other women to feel like they were not so alone. I hoped it would help them to make sure they got the help before they got as far into it as I did. I knew how lucky I was to get away with no real injuries and no real issues with my bone density, but I knew others would not be as fortunate.

I did, however, feel a little frustrated seeing the word "retired" in publications about my story; I didn't want to see it that way. It was scary to see it that way. Did I have to say I was never going to run seriously again? Couldn't I have both a running career AND a family if I was able to get my body back to health?

I do see how "*Elite runner stops running and gains weight to get menstrual cycles back and have baby, may one day return to elite running*" isn't exactly going to stop someone scrolling their social media, but did they really have to use that word: retire?

How old am I? 78?

The *Runners World* article was the one that really got things going, especially when it was shared by *Women's Health* magazine. I had some kickback on this one and as I didn't expect my story to go viral like it did, it hit me hard.

I am sensitive and tend to take comments to heart. I tried to remind myself that anyone who is trying to make a change in this world is going to come across people who do not agree with them. And that is okay! Not everyone is going to like you, but it is harder to ignore than it seems. After crying a little as I felt like I was being attacked for suggesting elite running=no period (which I certainly was not!), I did reflect and see how my words in *Runners World* could have come across as offensive without the rest of my story.

More than that though, I had to figure out a way to not let those comments get to me so much. If I was going to be a mother, I was going to have to learn to handle people being annoyed at me. No baby is going to allow you to sweet talk or reason your way out of a problem!

Some women can regulate their cycles and run high mileage with big intensity while maintaining a low weight, but I, and I am guessing you, are not one of those women. That makes it hard for us not to feel VERY jealous or even bitter towards the women who can get away with it, especially those who accidentally get pregnant while training hard.

Thousands of women have reached out to me since that day to say thanks for not making them feel so broken, which is exactly what I hoped for by sharing my story. I know how ashamed I felt that my body couldn't function correctly, and knowing you are not the only one can take a huge weight off your shoulders.

That is also where this book comes in. I wanted you to be able to have everything my brain knows about amenorrhea all in one place. I might not be an expert with a degree in biochemistry, but I can share with you my experience and what I have learned along the way.

Sharing my story has also sparked a greater conversation about this topic, which is good; it gets more awareness out there, and hopefully will mean more doctors and medical professionals can actually help us in future.

There will be a few sections with information from Dr. Nicola Rinaldi, author (along with coauthors, Stephanie Buckler and Lisa Sanfilippo Waddell) of the book _No Period. Now What?_ You will hear me reference this book a lot. It was an absolute game changer for me, and if you do not already have it, get it now!

It will be worth every penny, especially for the camaraderie you will feel from other women who have been in our situation. There is even a Facebook group, which is very helpful too.

I also have some sections with thoughts from the medical professionals who helped me through my journey: my endocrinologist, Dr. Wendell Miers and Harvard Sports dietitian Meg Steffey Shrier.

This book might not have all the science behind it, but it will have my experience and everything I have learned and did. You CAN overcome this, and you will, coming out the other side a much better person in every way. Let's see if we can build some confidence to show you that this is worth doing and you can get there.

My Story

As someone who got their first period a lot later than other girls in my class did, I was aware that my body was a little behind everyone else's from the start. I remember one of the boys in my class teasing me for being "flat-chested" around 14 and thinking it was the biggest insult in the world (although definitely true at the time), and I remember wondering why I wasn't having a period like all the other girls.

I wished for it, and when my period did arrive, I was relieved...in pain from cramps, but relieved I was "normal."

I don't really recall much else from those early days, other than having bowel movements a little more than usual during my period. I also remember the feeling of it dripping down once during an exam and hoping that it wouldn't show through my clothes.

I was growing into a woman, and that was all I cared about. My A-B bra was enough for me.

I started to lose my period again around age 17, when I made a big jump as a runner. I had quit horse riding to focus on my running and was driving two to three hours a week to train with Paula Radcliffe's (marathon world record holder) coach at Bedford and County Running Club.

We would run brutal sessions on the track, so hard I would fall to my hands and knees in exhaustion, but everyone was giving their best, so it just seemed normal. I have always had the ability to push myself hard, and at English running clubs, runners of all ages train together. You are not separated by age, but by ability. I was running alongside runners my age, mother runners, middle-aged runners, and everything in between. It didn't bother me; I just enjoyed having people to train with and a team atmosphere of working together to push the boundary of what was possible.

Looking back now, I am not sure the sessions were any harder than anyone else's training. I just felt the need to keep up with the other runners, even if they had years of running on me. Maybe I was pushing myself a little too hard those days, and that was part of the problem, especially as I was trying to juggle two running clubs: my sessions at Bedford, along with workouts with my coach back in Hertfordshire. I don't think I was overtraining; my mileage was still probably only around 30 miles a week, but the intensity increase, as someone who can push to the limit, was probably quite drastic.

I remember a few months going by without a menstrual cycle, so I talked to a few people about it. One of the coaches I knew suggested I take iron as low iron can often be linked to a lack of periods.

I began taking iron supplements the next day, not really seeing any harm with a little extra iron in my system. My period did soon return, and I was able to continue running as before...until the supplemental increase in iron began to catch up with my stomach, which was ripped to shreds by the iron tablets. I remember one workout where I had to run to the bathroom between every 400m repeat.

It was miserable.

I stopped taking the iron, but it seemed to have done the trick; my periods were back regular, and my running was going well.

One thing I do want to mention at this point is how thankful I am for my coach during my teenage years. If you have known me for a while, you have probably heard me talk about my former coach (and still mentor), Brad. Many girls were pushed very hard as teenagers, stretched to their limit, running higher mileage in a week than I did in a month, and most of them are no longer running. Exhausted both physically and emotionally, they ended up at a place where they despised running and would be lucky if they ever ran a 5k again.

I am so thankful that Brad was determined from the day I met him at age 14 that he wanted me to have a running CAREER, not just a fleeting few years while my body was still developing. Without Brad, I wouldn't be where I am today; I know that.

I carried on as usual for a few years, gaining a few pounds along the way as I went out to the clubs and pubs a little more than I probably should have and spent 8 months in California for a "gap year."

In England, it is pretty common to take a year off after school to travel and explore the world a little. I was enjoying my California girl life of frozen yogurt with a mountain of candy (it's yogurt, so it's healthy though, right?) and Panda Express (ick!). I wasn't overweight, just a normal teenage girl. I continued to run, still running hard on some days, just maybe not as intensely as before.

The following fall, I had plans to go back to California to go to university there. Well, go to a community college and transfer to University of California, Irvine, once I did the entry exams (I decided I wanted to go to university in the US too late to get in to the bigger universities!).

However, the universe had other plans for me. My visa was denied, and I was stuck in England, deflated and depressed. Through some crazy twist of fate, I ended up being accepted for a US visa to go to Ferris State University in Michigan, VERY last minute, and I was unsure what I was getting myself into.

When I arrived in Michigan, I was pretty out of shape. I hadn't taken my running seriously in almost a year, and it was clear that college running is serious business. It is essentially a job. There are many perks, but you'd better be ready to work hard and do your part. When you are brought over to the US on a full ride, you have even more expectation on your shoulders. I was definitely feeling the pressure.

I arrived at Ferris State wanting to be top dog. I was initially put in my place, falling behind and struggling to keep up with the other girls. My chin about fell to the floor when they informed me I would soon start running seven days a week. I was horrified! What sicko runs EVERY day of the week? (Now I laugh at that; most of my elite career I ran seven days a week, sometimes twice a day!)

I rose to the challenge, and began to do whatever I could to get better. I knew I had a long road ahead to get to my potential and I was far from my previous racing shape, but I was determined to get there.

One day, I remember overhearing a coach (who no longer coaches, FYI), telling another girl on the team that she would run faster if she lost 10lbs. I furrowed my brow in confusion.

Why would that help?

I had seen many very thin girls in my running career. I remember being on the bus to races while I was in school, and seeing girls eat basically nothing before races. I thought to myself that they were weird for not eating, how could you run fast without eating?

I just ignored their strange habits and carried on eating my pasta, grapes, chicken, and mayonnaise (do not ask me where the heck that came from, but that was my pre race meal...that or peas, butter and rice!). Those girls I had seen barely eating had flash-in-the pan careers and I didn't want to end up like them, so I continued to eat whatever I wanted when I wanted.

On this day though, I turned the comment I had just heard the coach make to myself. Looking down at my body, I wondered, was I overweight too?

I asked the coach later that day if I would do better losing some weight, to which he replied, "Yes." I don't remember his exact response, but what happened next could have been a dangerous spiral.

I started to limit my caloric intake, not drastically, as I have never been able to resist food and a buffet style cafeteria makes it difficult to not eat, especially for a college student who is hungry from training. I definitely started trying to make "better decisions" though. I lost a little weight towards the end of the year and my times started to improve with it, not because of the weight loss, but because the fitness was finally coming together.

As I went into my summer training, there was a coaching changeover and I knew things would be different going into my sophomore year. The change in my mindset had already started to take effect, though. I was building up to 50 miles per week while working two jobs as a waitress, meaning there was little energy to spare. I began to lean down, which secretly made me feel great as the words from the former coach still rattled around my brain. By this point, I was committed; I wanted to be faster.

Other girls on my team had also wanted to be faster and fitter, and looking back now, I wonder how many of them that previous coach had talked to. It became pretty easy to turn eating healthy into a competition; who could be best? Take a group of highly competitive, stubborn girls and there is almost no limit to how far you will go.

When we had our physicals on the first day back on campus, the trainers noted I had lost 12lbs since the last physical, and I knew that the 12lbs was definitely all in the second half of the year, particularly the summer. This made me feel a little happy, but still for me, at this point, it was all about the speed. I wanted to be faster.

I continued to train hard, and now, in the peak of cross-country season, this was the most intense training I had been through, but I wanted it, BAD.

It was around then I noticed I had been skipping a few periods. As it had worked before, I started to take iron pills again, but this time, it did not bring them back. It did bring the cramps back though. I was not prepared to poop my pants every time I ran to give it more time.

I didn't really think anything of it, it was too easy to brush off and push aside to deal with when I wasn't so "busy." I was having success in my running, my performances were skyrocketing, especially when I finished 12th at the Division II National Cross Country championships in November 2008.

Things were looking up, and I have to admit, I saw not having a period as a blessing. Not because I saw it as an accomplishment, but because it meant I didn't have to worry about trying to race on my period or carry around tampons. I could just get on with my training without any concerns about it.

Sometime early the next year, I had to go to the sports medicine doctor at Ferris for some kind of minor injury, and he asked me the typical question of, *"what was the date of your last period."* I looked down at the ground as I gave my answer; it had been a while. He noted it down and planted the seed in my mind that maybe this wasn't normal.

At the end of the school year, I decided I wanted to try to figure out what was wrong. Deep down I knew it wasn't healthy, and I have never been someone to take the easy way out for things.

I went to see an OB/GYN to make sure nothing was wrong internally; they did an ultrasound and bone density test, and found that everything was good. They said it was most likely the weight loss that caused my periods to stop and it should be a relatively easy fix.

I was given the Provera challenge, 10 days of progestin pills, which would hopefully kick start my cycles after the 10 days.

Nothing.

I was then put on a much stronger hormone, estropipate, for 21 days I believe, and another Provera challenge after, which hopefully would bring on the period.

This time it did work, except those few days of my menstrual cycle were incredibly painful. I was visiting home in England at the time, and had a friend from Ferris there with me. I remember crawling up into bed for a few days, feeling like someone was stabbing me in the uterus. To this day, I remember that being one of the most painful experiences of my life.

At least I knew everything was okay.

Unfortunately, that was not necessarily a good thing. It allowed me to just move on and forget about it. It became easy to brush it under the carpet and say it would come back when it was time. I was only 20, so really, what did it matter? I wasn't ready for kids anyway, and my running career was really showing some promise; why would I sabotage it now?

Around this time, the OB/GYN recommended I go on birth control (Loestrin) to make sure I continued to get the hormones. One of the side effects of birth control can be not having the bleeding each month, making it once again easy to dismiss.

I took my birth control and on I went with my running. Whenever the question of my last period came up, I would have an awkward few minutes of saying I didn't know, followed by a last ditch attempt to ask this particular physician about it, hoping he might have an answer as to what was going on, to which he would not. I would just move on with my day. Almost every doctor I saw would just say, *"It's probably just the running, all you need to do is stop running, and I am sure it will come back."*

Except that wasn't an option for me. Not only was I contracted to be a runner and Ferris State was paying for my entire college expense, but I didn't want to. Why would I give up running now to start again?

Once I told them that not running was not an option, they would essentially shrug their shoulders. As a three-sport athlete (cross-country, indoor track and outdoor track) you were training year round, other than a 1-2 week break twice a year; it was just not realistic.

Life carried on. I made an excuse to leave the room whenever girls would talk about their period symptoms and it became the new normal.

I achieved a lot, took significant jumps and ended up an 11 time Division II All American. I was proud of that, and had no intention of stopping there.

Once I started my masters at La Salle University, I became an assistant coach and mentor to college runners, who would often ask me personal questions as the only female coach for the team. I prayed they wouldn't ask me about how to run with period cramps or the diarrhea that comes with periods. It had been so long since I remembered those symptoms by this point.

Those questions of course did come, and they forced me to start thinking about the fact that I was not having a cycle. When the girls would tell me they were not having a cycle and ask what they could do to get it back, how could I tell them that it was not normal and healthy and they should get it figured out, when I too was ignoring the same issue?

One day while out on a long run with my friend Frances (Markowitz, née Koons) and a new friend she had introduced me to, Esther (Atkins, née Erb), we started talking about periods. Frances had a shorter run as a middle distance runner, and Esther and I had marathon long runs. During that run, I confided in Esther that I had not had a period in many years. She told me about how she had lost her cycle in the past too, but it had coincided with coming off birth control. After some time, she got her cycles back.

For the first time in many years, after endless amounts of doctors just saying to *"stop running,"* I felt excited. I felt that maybe I had my answer. I had long forgotten that I wasn't on birth control when they originally stopped!

So I stopped taking birth control and waited...and waited...and waited.

It can take up to a year, Esther said, so I held on to a little beacon of hope, even though I knew deep down my problem was more than just birth control.

After a year, I knew that I obviously was not in the same situation as Esther, and it really began to affect me. I was determined to figure this out somehow.

Thankfully, at this point, Sarah (Crouch, née Porter) had started a Facebook message about contraception and how it affected performance with at least 50 elite or professional runners. Many of them were absolute idols of mine, and I could barely believe I was in a conversation with them talking about such a personal subject.

It turned into a conversation about menstrual cycles and how common they were, asking advice for how to deal with them. Many of the girls also confessed to not having a cycle, which reassured me, while igniting that fire in me to do something about it.

The main suggestions were to increase your fat intake and eat more calories overall, and with that you would be able to maintain your cycle, regardless of size or weight. This frustrated me a little, as many of the runners in there were significantly thinner than I was, and I knew I ate well. I hadn't really restricted myself from calories, so why was this happening to me?

I began researching it a little more, trying to increase my fat intake as well as overall calories, but well into marathon training by this point, I was not exactly gaining weight.

Once I began as the podcast host for *Runners Connect*, I was introduced to Tawnee Gibson (née Prazak), the host of the *Endurance Planet* podcast. I wanted to bring her on *Run to the Top* to have her share her wisdom with my audience. As Tawnee began to share stories from her life, she talked about amenorrhea, the loss of menstrual cycles, and how it had taken her years to regulate her period. As Tawnee talked about how she used to be, the personality traits, the habits, how stressed she was about being successful in everything she did, it just hit me in the gut.

Everything she was saying about her life at that time was me in that moment. I was doing exactly what she had been doing: thinking more training was better, more activities were better, getting up earlier was better. The more things you could juggle in one go, the more successful you were, except there was a price to pay, and I had been paying it since 2008. My body was NOT in a healthy place.

The podcast with Tawnee was a real wake-up call for me. It made me want to cry as I finally realized that my body had been screaming for help all this time. I was determined to do something about it, and at this point, I was going to do everything I could to fix it...except give up running. I wanted to be healthy, but I also had many major running goals I still wanted to achieve, and I wasn't going to give up now after all those years of working to build my fitness year after year.

How could others get away with harder training, eating less, and pushing themselves more than I, yet I was the one who was unable to have a fully functioning body? I was careful to get many healthy foods in, yes, including fats, and I made sure I ate enough...my sweet tooth made sure I ate enough.

It was frustrating, and it didn't seem fair.

I began to dig. I confided in Tawnee about my struggles. As we traded stories, it felt like we were sisters; as she was talking about various things in her life, I felt like she was describing my life. It was almost eerie, and we began to call one another twin.

Regardless, I was just happy I had found someone else who understood, someone else who had been in a similar situation and come out the other side.

I knew Tawnee did consulting for athletes, and although Steve and I were trying really hard to save money, I knew it was worth investing. Tawnee had done a lot of work on health from a holistic standpoint, and I wanted to pass the reins over to someone who really "got it." I admired her, and I really liked her; it was worth the try.

We did a few phone calls; she looked into my nutrition, doing yet another food log, but once again finding that I was eating enough. She introduced me to some other experts in the field, but more holistic wellbeing professionals, where I met Chris of *Nourish. Balance. Thrive.* Chris suggested I take a DUTCH analysis of urine, which was much more accurate than a blood test to give me a hormonal status.

I did the test, but unsurprisingly at this point, he came back with "everything looks good." Not that there's anything wrong with the DUTCH test, it is very helpful for a variety of situations and I am glad I did it, but there wasn't really anything glaringly obvious in there to give an answer as to what was happening.

Tawnee and I continued to talk, and she suggested I cut back on the running. She thought it would be best if I could make sure my heart rate stayed in MAF zone (I will explain what that is later), and cut my volume of miles drastically. She also wanted me to reduce the empty carbs and junk food, replacing them with more fats and proteins along with high-quality nutrient carbs. I could do the nutritional changes, but for me, the running was non-negotiable. I didn't see the point in running if I was going to lose a lot of fitness and essentially, my elite level running. I wanted to try the other things first, see if I could get it back with the nutrition changes.

So I did.

I ended up a somewhat high fat, high protein, low carb runner. Not through any fault of Tawnee's, I just wasn't getting enough carbs for my volume of training. I was still having higher carbs than an average person, but for a runner, it was definitely in the low carb zone. I was eating avocados galore, coconut butter by the spoonful out of the jar, four egg omelets, and all the vegetables you can imagine. My food prep on a Sunday involved trays upon trays of roasted vegetables to consume throughout the week, all roasted up nicely in butter or ghee.

Tawnee also pushed for me to cut out the sugar, well, in excess. I had always eaten sweets every few hours throughout the day: a handful of M&Ms here, a few Twizzlers there, and then a big dessert every single evening, a bowl of ice cream or a giant cookie. That was just life for me. My mum has always been a big sweets eater, as has my grandma (notorious for going out for lunch and having a cake for her lunch and a different cake for her "pudding" (dessert for Americans!).

Cutting out sweets was not only impossible for me, but I had done it before in college and was miserable. I enjoyed eating sweets and yes, sad to say, it brought me happiness to do so.

I agreed to cut down, to have the dessert in the evening and try to limit the sweets during the day. Tawnee had a theory that I was basically running on sugar, which was leaving my body in a high alert state.

I tried really hard on the diet changes, all while my training ramped up. I actually ended up completing my major life goal during this time: representing Great Britain and Northern Ireland in the World Half Marathon Championships, and then five weeks later running a four-minute PR, and for the first time running under 2:40 (a big time goal for me) in the marathon while this was happening.

When I stayed with my parents for 5 weeks between those races, I was very strict with what I needed to eat. I would turn my nose up at non-organic food; I would scoff at people eating bread. I definitely became a food snob, and I would say I edged on orthorexic...of course except for the sweets.

I still needed them every day.

In fact, I felt I couldn't go to bed without having something. I always said that if I was in the middle of nowhere and I hadn't had my sweets by 9pm that night, I would go out wandering until I found a gas station to get a bar of chocolate. If I went to bed without my dessert, it would bother me, like really make me feel like a part of me was missing, and I had insane cravings for it.

I still believe to this day that although extreme in many ways, my sweet tooth saved me from becoming orthorexic; I still loved my dessert, and I was not going to give it up. When we talk to experts or consultants, most of us feel scared to say what we really mean, promising them we will do our best, when really, we are kind of smiling and nodding so they don't judge us. For me, while consulting with Tawnee, I stood my ground; cutting out the sweets was a hard no and I was prepared to fight for it. It was not realistic for me to cut them out completely, nor did I want to.

I ran some of the defining races of my career during this phase, and I was feeling strong. I looked lean, I was fit, I was healthy, and I felt really good. I didn't have the mental haze in long runs anymore; I felt like I was full of energy and not craving food all the time. I didn't really miss the typical "stodgy carbs" as I called them then: bread, pasta, oatmeal, and I genuinely loved eating all the food that I knew was making my body feel good.

I had regular Inside Tracker tests (you can use code TINAMUIR for 10% off) to look at my blood work, and it came up with optimal results in most things, other than that my cholesterol had gone up, unsurprisingly from the amount of meat I was now eating, and my DHEAS were very low, but that wasn't different to any other blood test I had in the past.

The main thing though, I still had no period, not even a sign of it.

I would cling on to the hope that maybe it was coming back when I would look in my underwear and see some kind of change in the cervical fluids.

But it never came.

I went to see an endocrinologist to see if we could find anything there. I wanted to dive deeper into my hormones as this was ultimately what decided whether I would menstruate or not, and an endocrinologist was the next level of expert I thought might have an answer. I had talked to Neely (Gracey) about amenorrhea in the past, and she said the endocrinologist noticed her issue and was able to solve it right away.

I was hopeful as I walked into the office of Dr. Wendell Miers; maybe my issue was the same thing as Neely's and it would be a simple solution; half a pill a week would fix things for good.

Unfortunately, this was not the case, but Dr. Miers really did seem to understand what running meant to me. He was a runner and I felt like I had hit the jackpot because although he was not a woman, he got it. He saw how "just stopping" is not as easy as it sounds to non runners, and he told me that my hormone levels showed that I was close, just not quite there. He was confident that I would get my cycles back within 3-6 months of cutting back on the running and increasing my caloric intake.

Although it wasn't the answer I wanted, although I wasn't ready to accept that fate, Dr. Miers did have a big impact on my journey. He was the first medical professional who gave me hope and really seemed to care, and was prepared to give me a timeline of how long he thought it would take to get things back on track. Once I said I would not stop running to every other medical professional, they had essentially pushed me aside and said, *"Well, I can't help you."*

I was thankful that at last I had found a runner who knew what it meant to me, and who gave me hope that this didn't mean no running forever. I just had to get things going again, and I would be able to figure out how running would fit into my life after I had regained my cycles.

Later that summer, I was doing a speed segment in my training, which meant faster workouts on the track, and shorter races. I noticed that I was having a hard time getting my speed up. It had not clicked together as it had before, and I was really struggling.

I blamed it on the heat and humidity. I blamed it on too much going on in my life. I blamed it on anything and everything except things I ultimately had control over. All of this while noticing this little voice in my head that would pop up from time to time questioning why I even bothered.

Of course we all have that thought in races (yep, elites too), we wonder why we put ourselves through this when sitting on the couch watching TV sounds so much more appealing, but those thoughts are usually fleeting. Those thoughts usually show up when you are really pushing yourself hard. Now they were appearing at random times, and I was finding it a lot harder to push myself hard without my inner dialogue encouraging me to slow down or even stop.

After a terrible race at Falmouth, I decided it was time to step back and reflect. Something was going on here. Falmouth should have been a good race for me. It was humid and hot, it was hilly, and it was tough competition, but I usually thrive on those conditions. Instead, I barely made it at my tempo pace.

After some reflection, I realized I had taken my nutritional changes too far. I had ended up low carb, with most of my carbs coming from vegetables (which don't provide much) and my beloved desserts. But most runners REALLY struggle to run fast on a low carb diet. The night before Falmouth, I was so anti-pasta that I had a big salad with meat sauce on top.

Not exactly a pre-race meal.

I started to add carbs back into my diet, and took some time off, noticing that I was feeling better. My period had not returned, so it was not like that aspect of me was now working. I still kept a lot of the good stuff I was eating daily, like the massive amounts of vegetables and fats, but just added back a lot more carbs.

I raced California International Marathon in December of that year feeling good. I trained hard, my mind was mostly in a good place, personal life events had calmed down, and I felt like I had turned the corner from those thoughts earlier in the year. They still appeared from time to time, but like before, I could push them out.

I ran a one-minute PR at CIM, which actually was a bit of a disappointment as every other marathon I had done, I had shaved four minutes off. Ungrateful? Yes, maybe, but it wasn't like I hadn't worked for them. I felt like I was better than the 2:36 next to my name, but coming in those final miles, my quads were just shot. I had nothing left to give, so I was proud of my effort.

This is where life really began to change.

Returning to running after my usual 10 days off exercise was more of a struggle than usual. I noticed that my body still felt tired and sore...not really too surprising, considering the downhills early in the race really beat my body up. I tried not to become discouraged.

Another month went by, and I still didn't feel like myself. I was going back and forth with the race director of Gold Coast Marathon, the next race I wanted to do in July. I knew I had plenty of time, but it was hard not knowing where I was going next, what I was training for (which is ironic now, as I really enjoyed a 2018 without any kind of goal!) I struggled with that, but just did the best I could for the time being.

There was a bigger problem though; the negative voice was back, and showing up more than ever. It told me that I didn't want to do this anymore. It was there early whispering in my ear during easy runs, long runs, workouts, before it even got hard.

I found myself struggling to want to push, dreading workouts, and just feeling very blasé about running. The best word to describe my thoughts towards running in this time was UGH.

On February 2 2017, my niece Charlotte was born. I remember that moment so clearly. Finishing my warmup for a workout at Cold Stream Park, now knowing officially that I was going to be racing the Gold Coast marathon on July 2. I had even announced it to the world a few weeks prior. I was so excited for this race, but at the same time, still didn't quite feel right. I also had an added pressure of agreeing to pace the 2:28 group for the London Marathon. I was expected to go 1:14 for a half marathon in April. Running 5:38 per mile for 13 miles seemed like an almighty task. I knew I had done it before, but for some reason, things weren't coming together as they had in the past.

Anyway, back to that day:

I remember going back to the car to change my shoes, and receiving a call from my mum telling me my sister was in labor. I found it even harder than my new normal (of struggling) to motivate myself. I felt on edge and just wanted it to be over so I could get back to the car. I knew labor might take a while, but I wanted to be with my family so desperately.

After the workout, I went right to my strength training session with Drew. We were not even 10 minutes into the workout when I got the call. I had a baby niece, and mama was healthy as well.

I fell to the ground crying tears of joy. It was the most incredible feeling. I was so proud of my sister, so excited to meet this new little person, and suddenly felt so very far away. ALL I wanted to do was to be there in that hospital with my family, congratulating my beloved sister on bringing life into this world. It was my first experience of suddenly feeling a love for someone you have never known, but who leaps straight into your heart.

I booked a flight, and headed to England when Charlotte was two weeks old. I was obsessed with her and held her any minute I could. Just appreciating being still with her, listening to her little breaths, and feeling her warmth.

My sister's husband is a pediatric nurse, meaning he often works nights. Although he had a few weeks off before he had to go back to work, he did have shifts while I was still in England. That meant I spent nights with my sister and her 4-week-old baby, who was having a hard time feeding and sleeping (we later found out because of a tongue-tie). I helped the best I could.

Every few hours in the night, Charlotte would cry and need a feed. After her feed, we would spend 40 minutes trying to settle her. Two hours later, the cycle would start again. I was trying to be as supportive as I could be without overstepping my boundaries. But it was hard, really hard.

I have always put my family before my training. I might ask them to move things around slightly, but I would drop my running in a second if my family really needed me. During this time, I felt serious anxiety around my training. With barely any sleep, trying to run 90 miles a week with workouts meant I was living in a state of stress and fear. The sleep deprivation meant that I was not only feeling physically tired, but it also made that negative voice even louder in my ear.

Done. Done. Done. Was what it said to me, over and over.

I could see this new little person just trying to survive, just trying to make it through the day. My sister, exhausted and sleep deprived. Here was me, out running for multiple hours a day. For what? I had achieved my biggest goal. I had accomplished many things I could be very proud of, but there was so much more to life.

Was this really the life I wanted anymore?

During my visit home, I had an appointment with someone I hoped might give me some answers about why I was dealing with amenorrhea. I had booked the appointment six months in advance to see a naturopath named Natasha whom my aunt had seen a few times a year for many years. My auntie, Jenny, has a blood cancer, which Natasha is treating alongside her hematology doctor. Natasha is a Heilpraktiker, homeopath, electro-acupuncturist and microbiologist (phew! That is quite a title!). She does not have a website, and answers the phone for one hour a day...if you can even get through, which I was never able to.

I was skeptical, but at this point, prepared to try it.

I drove the one hour from my parents' house to the absolute middle of nowhere, a house located in the countryside. I parked in the driveway and sat in what is I guess a waiting room. There was no one to greet me, no one around other than a young child just playing. The child would come over to me from time to time, show me a drawing or talk to me about whatever she saw. I did not know whom the child belonged to, or when it was going to be my turn to go in.

I was essentially sitting in a living room, and around half an hour after my appointment time passed, I heard noises coming from a different room, and saw a couple walk by with a white bag of clinking bottles.

Natasha came out of the room a few minutes later, and was everything I expected of a naturopath. She was a little out there, but absolutely lovely. Taking me back to what seemed to be a messy office combined with some kind of science lab. Natasha did electrodermal screening, which does seem a little woo-woo, even for me, but part of me was excited to see what she found.

Unfortunately (or fortunately), Natasha told me I was one of very few she has ever seen who was in genuinely good health. She did find a few little things I had going on that could be worked on, and I told her about the lack of menstruation, which she gave me drops to help with. She wanted me to go see her again at Christmas if my cycle had not resumed, although she wasn't sure it would work. I did what I was told and took my drops for the next few weeks until they were gone. I saw Natasha two weeks before I stopped running (if that), so I will never really know how much of a role the drops played.

I talked to a few family members and friends about my feelings, who mostly just reminded me that they were there for me, they still loved me no matter what I chose, and that it was okay to not love running anymore. Honestly, most of them who are not runners and have never been runners, were probably feeling relieved, *FINALLY she will be able to not live her life around this sport.*

One friend, Kat, who had been a runner in her past, a very good one actually, had stopped running in her late teens because of a rare mitochondrial disease that made running pretty much impossible for her body. As a former Great Britain and Northern Ireland athlete as a teenager, I knew she would get the significance of this. I was there for her during her tough transition out of the sport, and she had since found a passion for singing, playing in a band, and songwriting. She is very good at it, making a career out of it actually, and maybe she wouldn't have discovered that without stopping running. That gave me hope that without running, maybe I too, could find something else to enjoy and do.

Kat reminded me that I could always stop running and restart. There was nothing saying that I couldn't get a month in and change my mind. Sure, I would have lost a bit of fitness, but I could just pretend it was an injury, and it would come back quickly. We all know deep down that running fitness comes back fast (even though it may not feel like it at the time!).

That helped with the mental side, knowing I could in fact go back at any point I wanted to. Prior to the conversation with Kat, it was hard to not see it as black and white. Keep running or be done forever.

The voice telling me to stop, quit, why bother, got louder and louder. It was soon on every run with me, from start to finish. As I had pain in my anterior tibialis, it gave me yet another reason to hate it. Every step hurt, every mile I wished I was done, every two a day I dreaded.

Until one day, I snapped.

I have been interviewed hundreds of times in my years as a professional athlete. One of the first questions that's asked is about how I started running. When did I become interested, and how did I decide to be a runner?

I do not remember my first experience running; I do not remember when I first joined the cross-country team or my first race.

What I do remember is running around Westminster Lodge fields in my hometown of St Albans for many of my races, and then running around the track. Both with a brilliant view of the St Albans Cathedral, our proudest attraction, and our best representation of what our city has to offer.

It's somewhat ironic that 14 years later, it would be that same view that would be in my line of vision as I finally decided it was time to step away.

The morning I was leaving to go back to the US, March 21 2017, I had a track workout to do early in the morning. I headed over to the track before it was open, and jumped the fence (just a small fence, before you go thinking of me scaling barbed wire!). I had done this before, and figured no one would notice. It was probably 6:30am, not exactly prime time.

I think I had about 6 x 800 to do, something along those lines...as you will read in a minute, I didn't end up recording it. There I was, going through the first few reps, trying my hardest to ignore that voice telling me that I didn't want this kind of runner life anymore, when one of the staff from the Westminster Lodge track storms across the track towards me. He yells, "YOU CAN'T BE OUT HERE." I told him I had to finish my rep (I had 100m to go), and then I would be back over to him.

I jogged over to him, and tried to explain that I was an elite runner, I was working with Everyone Active (the gym on site), and that I only had a few 800s to go, I would be done in 15 minutes max.

He was not having it.

He told me I had to leave right now, I was not allowed on this track. I tried one last ditch attempt to reason with him, telling him that the local paper was doing an article on me that day, about how I was an Olympic hopeful and I was training hard to prepare for my upcoming race. Surely, it would look good for them that I was training on their track?

Nope.

So I walked off the track, crying, and then just stopped in my tracks.

I'm done.

Usually in this situation, I would have been flustered; I would have probably gone much slower in those final few repeats, doing my best with the surrounding area to finish what I needed to do. I would have replayed what just happened over and over again, as I tried to wrap my head around it. There were paths and flat areas nearby to finish if I wanted to, ironically, the place where my running began. The cross-country course where I first recognized my competitiveness and desire to run. I had so many memories in this park, on that track I was just removed from, and here I was, it had all come down to this. Being kicked off and unable to continue, both physically and emotionally.

There had to be some level of symbolism with that moment.

I was done.

Fed up with running. Fed up with hearing that voice telling me to quit.

I give in, you win.

I felt broken, weak, and defeated.

Unfortunately, I was still 2.5 miles from my house, which meant I had no choice but to run home. I had no phone or any way to get back without doing the one thing I refused to do.

My pride would not allow me to ask someone to use their phone and get someone to pick me up, mostly because it was early in the morning, and by now the rush hour traffic would be strong. It would take my dad longer to get to me than it would to run home. I just wanted to be done.

I didn't even bother to restart my watch; I just began to run, blubbering as I went. Feeling so sorry for myself and hating everything about what I was doing. I was essentially mourning my running career. I felt like I was breaking up with a boyfriend, knowing we were wrong for each other, but just trying to get through that initial heartbreak of knowing it is over.

At one point along the path (thankfully, I could run the back way home, so although I saw many people out walking, I was shielded from cars), I saw a blonde girl up ahead. I hoped and prayed it was my friend Keeley, another runner, who actually had a baby less than 2 months after I did!

I just wanted a hug.

As the girl moved closer, I realized it was not Keeley, and I just had to keep going, hyperventilating in that unique way only girls and babies know how.

When I finally arrived home, I was still crying. I knocked on the door and my dad opened it. I fell onto the hallway floor and just cried. Cried and cried and cried.

"I'm done," was all I could say.

By this point, my sister and Charlotte had come around the corner, up early to come say goodbye to me before I went. As they looked at me curled up in the hallway, I felt my heart breaking. Not only did I now have to go through this breakup, but I only had my family for a few precious minutes before I had to leave them, a part of my life that still crushes me every time.

My mum, dad, and sister didn't really know what to say, at a loss for words for how to comfort me, none of them being runners, and my mum now having to leave for work or she would be late. I picked up the phone and began to call Steve; it was 2am in Kentucky, but I didn't care. I figured he needed to hear this.

He answered, panicked; wondering what could possibly be going on for me to call at this time when I would see him later that day.

"I'm done," I kept repeating over and over. Crying through the phone.

He told me that he would see me soon, we would talk about it and figure out where to go from here. At the time, I am not sure he knew how serious I was, but either way, at least he knew.

I traveled back to the US, having all those hours on the flight to mourn my running career and think about where I wanted to go now.

Of course, I knew I could always go back to running and I do strongly believe I will be one of those women who come back stronger as she gets older.

But it wasn't about that. It was more about the decision to give in.

As runners, we pride ourselves on being strong, tough, and gritty. I saw stopping running as a way to quit, and I am not a quitter. I also felt guilt about wasting my talent.

I am very fortunate to have been given this ability to run fast, and combined with the hard work I have put in over the years, it has allowed me to solidify myself as one of Great Britain's best runners.

Isn't it a waste to throw that away? Will I look back on myself at age 28 and wonder why I didn't give it a few more years to really see what I could do?

And why would you quit while you're ahead?

I had run a PB in every marathon I had completed, and my improvements over the years showed strong and steady progress. Stepping away should be done when you have accomplished all your hopes and dreams, and you are satisfied with all you have done. I know I had more in there for all the main distances from 5 k marathon.

Here are some words I wrote to myself while 35,000 feet in the air:

The last few months, I have felt different in a way I can't describe. I feel broken, beaten, and devastated.

I haven't had a major injury, but I found myself almost wishing that something big would come up. Something that would make the decision for me, and show me that it was time to shift my focus on a family, rather than myself. But this isn't just about me. This is about my husband too, that wonderful man who has given up countless hours of his time to help me realize those dreams.

Who am I to throw that all away when I am only 28 years old?

No big injury did arise. No decision was made for me.

All I had was relentlessly tight calves, making every run a little painful. Not unbearable, but definitely uncomfortable and then there were the workouts.

We did take a little more time down after CIM than in the past. Not more time off as in days of no running, but we took the return to running a little slower than usual, my request as I was feeling so beaten up from the course. Maybe this was my intuition quietly tapping me on the shoulder, reminding me that it is okay to take a break.

For a few weeks, things were going well. I knew I had lost fitness, but I felt excited about the future. I did struggle with focus and motivation without knowing what my next goal race was. As we waited for the Gold Coast Marathon to let me know their plans, I found myself having more trouble in workouts. The easy runs were okay, but the workouts were not going as well as I had hoped.

But once we did confirm that Gold Coast was the next marathon for me, I thought YES, this is finally going to kick me back into shape. I am excited about the race. This is the opportunity of a lifetime, and I am going to make the most of it.

But GCAM was so far away, that it was easy to slip back into my mindset of having plenty of time. My nutrition wasn't as good as it should be. I found myself often telling myself about living life rather than looking after my body as best I could to run to my potential. The little details that had always mattered and made the difference on race day were now inconveniences that grated me.

Once I added the London marathon pacing in there, this added a pressure that I could not remove. I was always boasting about how good I was at pacing, and now I really had the opportunity to prove it, with the best runners in Great Britain relying on me to do my job correctly.

Over the coming months, the harder I tried to get my training in, the more I found I was struggling. My workouts began to go downhill, and although I was giving my best, doing all I can, just like I tell everyone else, I found that my heart was falling out of love with running. It became about getting it done, rather than enjoying the process. They started to get slower and slower, and I found the voice telling me to stop getting louder and louder. Until this morning, when the voice became so loud that I did slow to a walk.

Done.

I know that running is a huge part of my life, and I love the sport. I love that what you put in is what you get out, and I mentioned that last year at CIM I almost think I didn't run as well because I didn't have any setbacks, I always run the best after overcoming setbacks.

This is not just a setback anymore. This is a screaming voice telling me that I need to quit.

I tried to push the voice out, and once I reached the point where I was far enough into the workout to just focus on surviving the next minute, I could. I was able to get back into my usual mindset of just giving my all, but I knew that the next day the voice would be back.

After 14 years of this being my life, it is not so easy to stop, even if you know it is the right thing to do. I know in my heart it is time for the next era of my life. I have moved on from my job at RunnersConnect, I have had the time at home to remind me what is really important in life, and I have all the signs that show me its time.

But after all those years of being in that same cycle; train, race, rest, rebuild. Repeat.

The idea of stepping out of that comfort zone and really being forced to face who I really am, what I really am, is *f*cking terrifying. Running has given me so much; it has given me so many opportunities, connections, experiences.*

What if no one is interested in me anymore without my credentials?

I still love it, I still want to be involved in it, and this doesn't change anything about running for Real and my business. This is the ultimate real factor isn't it? I am admitting that I am not in love with running right now, my own running anyway. What really makes me happy is making other people happy, and that is what I can do from my business, regardless of whether I run or not.

The reality is, I have to have more than that in my life. I can give myself to my business, but then I will burn out in the same way. If I am going to do this, I am going to do it to start a family, and my situation is a little more complicated than most. It will require a few years of changes. It will require minimal activity; it will probably require gaining more weight. That is not an easy pill to swallow, but I tell people over and over again to love who they are, that they have so much more to offer the world, and maybe it's time I listen to my own advice.

I put that stream of consciousness aside as soon as I wrote it, and actually didn't go back to read it until I wrote this book. Now I can see my mind was already made up, but in the moment, I was still very much going back and forth.

I had to begin the journey of figuring out what my future looked like.

Without running, who was I? What did I want to be?

Something had clicked inside me seeing Charlotte. Not like a jealousy thing, because Jess was a mum and I wanted to be one, but more that having a child, bringing life into this world, was the one thing I wanted to do more than anything, it always had been.

If I didn't have running, if I didn't have that excuse for why my body isn't functioning correctly, I could go figure it out, finally.

As much as the prior few weeks of sleep deprivation, a screaming baby, and stress had been hard, I felt confident that I could do it. I could be a mother, and yes, I was ready for it now.

When I returned home, Steve and I went for a walk to talk about it. I tried…maybe even pleaded with him to tell me what he thought I should do. I had this huge opportunity of an expenses paid trip to the Gold Coast in Australia. Steve and I had said I would take one last attempt at the Commonwealth Games the following year (which would be raced on the same Gold Coast Marathon course), and then we would decide what to do about children.

Here I was, stopping over a year early and throwing away this opportunity.

Was it worth it? Was this just a slump I should push through? Take a week off, then try, try again?

As hard as I tried, Steve would not give me an answer. At the time, I felt frustrated with him for not helping me with my decision, but now, looking back, I realize it was 100% the right thing to do.

It HAD to be my choice.

Of course, a part of him would be sad that he would not be coaching me for this next race. He had told me that he really thought I was ready for a big breakthrough; I could be ready for a 2:32-ish marathon, which would be a HUGE step up in the elite world. However, he was also my husband, and he knew he wanted kids, so it would be okay if I chose the other option too.

We set a week to think about it. No running, but time for me to really look into my heart to see what I wanted. Steve was actually gone most of the week, as was I, taking a few of his athletes down to a meet in Raleigh, North Carolina, as I was Steve's only assistant coach at Morehead State at the time. I was distracted with tasks for his best athletes, although I did have time to read *The Mindset Manifesto* by Dr. Bhrett McCabe for an upcoming interview with him (now one of my most popular podcasts of all time).

I noticed as I was reading that the words were so inspiring, they should have encouraged change. I knew what they were trying to say, and any previous version of me would have been motivated after reading them, just as my listeners were after they heard the podcast episode. The words had no effect though, in one ear and out the other. I just didn't want it anymore. Nor did being at a track meet watching people run big personal bests and run-around with a smile motivate me. It just didn't make me want it at all.

I knew my answer.

I think I will always remember the moment I told Steve that I really did want to step away from running; I did want to try for a family. We were sitting at another track meet, the one he went to while I was in Raleigh. After the Raleigh Relays were complete, I drove the athletes I had with me to meet the rest of the team in Winthrop, South Carolina. We were sitting on the grass, and I told him I had made my decision, refusing to look at him, picking at the dead grass around the track to avoid eye contact.

I want to start our family. Now.

He was happy and excited with my decision. Not the ideal place to have that conversation, but this was it, we were going to do it, and that was all that mattered!

I immediately began to research. Anything and everything I could find on getting my period back, I was all over it. I had already purchased _No Period. Now What?_ the year before, now I could actually read it. At the time, I wasn't really ready for what they were telling me to do, so I had just put it aside.

Now I could devour it and as they call it, go "all in." The women in the book seemed to describe everything I was feeling word for word, and now I was committed, I had tunnel vision about it. Nothing else seemed to matter; I was going to get my period back as quickly as I possibly could. I was going to be the best damn period-get-backer there ever was.

The first opportunity I had, I booked an appointment at Lexington Women's Health with the OB/GYN I had seen a few years ago, who had told me, like every other medical professional, that whenever I was ready to stop running, she would be ready to help.

At the time, I felt frustrated by her response, but something told me that she was the right person to work with. I really liked Dr. Jennifer Fuson as a person, and I felt I could trust her with this next big step. The words of Dr. Miers, the endocrinologist I had seen about a year prior, stayed in the front of my mind. I could do 3-6 months... I was going to make sure it was on the three-month end, but that was manageable for me. I looked at things optimistically while I waited for my appointment to see Dr. Fuson.

All that was left to do, was it.

Follow through with my intentions and listen to the recommendations in _No Period. Now What?_ , which was the best source of information I could find, especially as Dr. Nicola Rinaldi was the only one who seemed to actually understand amenorrhea, and understand how difficult it would be for people like me (and you!) to actually make a change like they were suggesting.

I had somewhat of a step-by-step guide, and some other women who had been through it, to convince myself I was doing the right thing, that it would be worth it.

I had already started the rest aspect. I had already stopped running and exercising for my body to heal, and actually, I was enjoying it a lot more than I thought I would. I quickly filled the time with other activities, using this time to work on relationships and my business, which ironically, was called "Running for Real." Here I was, not running, but giving others advice on how to do so.

At this point, I had not yet told the world what was going on. That part of me did feel like a little bit of a fraud, like I was being deceitful, but I knew I didn't have to wait much longer to get that weight off my shoulders now we had committed.

I knew nutrition was a huge component of my recovery, and I had nothing to lose. If I was going to do it, I was going to do it right. There was no point putting in a half effort for this. What would be the point of resting and letting my muscles totally fade away, if I was not going to address another of the keys to getting my cycle back: gaining weight?

For the next four weeks, every time I was hungry, I ate. Even if that meant I was eating again one hour after the previous meal. Even if that meant eating late at night, even if that meant out- eating my husband. I figured the quicker I could gain weight; get my BMI well into the "normal" level, the better. The research I had done had suggested the 22-25 BMI range was ideal, which for me, at 18-19 BMI, didn't seem too hard. I felt like 15-20lbs did not seem life changing.

In the first few weeks, I often ate when I wasn't hungry; I just knew it would help with my cause, and while I could get away with it, why not make the most of it; I love to eat!

Once I opened the floodgates of eating whatever and whenever I wanted, I just became hungrier and hungrier. I was eating constantly. I decided early that if I was going to do this, I was going to make it as fun as possible. I made the best of it: GIANT ice cream bowls, peanut butter chocolate chip pancakes, fried chicken and fries. Not the healthiest diet in the world by a long shot, but I really enjoyed the freedom of just having whatever I felt like in the moment, rather than what I thought was best for my running or what I thought I "should" have.

I knew I would get back to eating nutritionally dense foods, but this was like a little vacation for my body, and I knew it would come to an end.

After another week of eating pretty much everything in sight, I decided it was time to tell the world about what was going on.

Okay, maybe not the world, I had no idea it was going to blow up the way it did, but I knew there were other women out there like me (like you!) going through this, and I wanted to show them they were not alone. I had a pretty loyal following of fans, and I felt like I was being deceptive by not telling them I had not only stopped running, but what was going on.

In typical Tina fashion, I poured my heart out onto a blog post. Sharing all my inner thoughts about what was going on, leaving it all out there, and really, opening myself up to criticism I did not anticipate. In that blog post, I declared that I was going to shout this from the rooftops; I was going to make sure people like you and I didn't feel like our bodies had failed us, as if we were the only ones who couldn't seem to function, as a woman should.

When I released the post on April 3 2017, it EXPLODED within the running community. My website crashed because it couldn't handle the volume of traffic. I think anyone and everyone who even knew my name was trying to read this monster post at the same time.

That day, I was traveling back home from a job interview for a brand in Boston (crazy now to think had I taken the job, I would have said "yes" to a job and a few weeks later told them I was pregnant and had to figure out what to do). I was in the airport, and happened to see a friend, Darren Brown, a pro triathlete, who was stuck in Atlanta too. After a hug hello, he told me his wife, Sarah Brown (also a professional runner), had texted him asking if he had seen my blog post (not knowing I was there). Darren had not read my blog yet, but he asked what the heck was going on; it would have to be something pretty big for Sarah to text him to ask.

After two weeks, 17,000 people had read that blog post, and I knew I had the leverage to get amenorrhea on the radar. I reached out to a friend, Ali Feller (*Ali on the Run*), who introduced me to an editor at *Runner's World*. They were immediately interested and I began writing my story. Writing for *Runners World* was much more difficult than writing my own blog post. By now, you can probably tell I am a total rambler, and cutting this story into 800-1000 words was not easy.

Which is where a lot of the criticism came in. My story became a little lost in translation. I made sure to recommend people read my entire blog post to get the full story, but we all know that unfortunately it doesn't always work like that.

When the story went out, I was nervous. I knew my family, friends, and fans would be supportive, but what about the rest of the world? They didn't know or care about me. It would bring all the trolls out of the woodwork, and I also knew that many people would wonder why this was even a conversation. This was something that should be kept private.

Well, turned out it did do well. Women from all over the world started to reach out to me from every place imaginable. I had literally THOUSANDS of emails and messages from other women saying they too were going through this. Other outlets began to pick it up: *SELF*, *Well+Good*, ESPN, *Outside Online*, *Women's Health*, *Glamour,* and of course, the one everyone notices, *People* magazine.

PEOPLE MAGAZINE!

I did not think I would ever end up in *People* magazine, and no, it wasn't the print version, but they ended up doing another two update posts on me. Which in itself was pretty comical, the first one was called, "Runner Who Started Gaining Weight 2 Months Ago to Get Period Back Says She Still Isn't Menstruating." I found that pretty funny! *People* also did one when I announced I was pregnant.

A strange feeling knowing that *People* magazine is watching you!

Once they picked it up, it spun even more out of control, and my phone was ringing off the hook for a while. I could barely keep up with the emails, and it was just crazy. However, at the same time, it was a nice distraction from what I was really doing: trying to get my period back.

If you had told me about this years ago, I would have thought all this conversation around me, all the podcasts, the interviews, would have put more pressure in the situation…making it less likely to actually happen. In fact, I really didn't feel that way. I mostly just felt support, especially from loved ones, but even more since I shared my story; I think people do try to be respectful of couples trying for a family, because we are now learning just how difficult it actually can be.

I held on to the words from Dr. Miers, my endocrinologist, but of course, being the stubborn runner, I wanted to do it in less time. If it was going to take most people four months, I wanted to do it in two, and by the time I got to around eight weeks, I began to feel frustrated that it had not happened yet.

It doesn't make sense.

I had done EVERYTHING I was supposed to do. I had gained 20lbs in 8 weeks. I had not exercised other than a few strength-training workouts after 6 weeks. I had gone for acupuncture. I was taking time each day to relax.

Why wasn't it working?

It felt like one of those moments in a movie. The one that comes to mind is Jim Carrey in *Bruce Almighty*, where he falls to his knees and yells to the sky. I was getting deflated and wondering why I even bothered at all.

Maybe I just wasn't meant to have kids.

So dramatic!

I purchased some ovulation sticks to reassure myself to stick with the plan. Not that I was considering starting to run again or losing the weight, I had come too far, but to at least know when things were going in the right direction, to keep a glimmer of hope. Particularly as I didn't know anyone personally who was going through this, whom I could talk to about it, and there wasn't a book like this to read the story of someone who knew how I felt. _No Period. Now What?_ had snippets of people's journeys, but not in enough detail to really help me feel connected to them (as I hope this book does for you!).

For the record, those ovulation sticks are a dangerous game. If you have struggled with calorie counting or have obsessive compulsive tendencies, I would recommend staying away from them as they might put more stress and pressure on the situation, which just puts your body back in that high alert state.

I knew these little sticks were cheap and unreliable. I knew I couldn't put too much into them, but at least then, maybe, I could see progress, that I was getting close to ovulating. I had read that after cessation of menstruation, your body may build up a few times with the hormones as it attempts to get things back on track. I thought those ovulation tests might show me that it was trying, maybe not quite ready yet, but getting close.

I reassured myself of this, and I did purchase three more expensive, accurate ovulation tests to use if I really did think I was ovulating. I knew ovulation was the best way to tell my period was on the way. If I was ovulating, my period WOULD be happening a few weeks later. The impatience in me taking over.

One day, I noticed a faint pink line next to the control line.

It was one of those lines where you can't really tell if it is a line, or if it is wishful thinking. I knew I had to wait until the next day, and I could barely wait until the following morning to pee on that stick. Not even telling Steve, as I was too embarrassed with how excited I was.

Sure enough, it was a little stronger the next day.

PROGRESS. YES!

But these lines have to be the same color to show ovulation.

It took a few more days, but then on May 17, not even two months after I stopped running, the lines were clearly the same color. Could I be?

I took the plunge of using one of the accurate Clearblue ovulation tests, and held my breath most of the five minutes. If it came up with a smiley face, I would indeed be ovulating, but if not, I knew I was close.

Surely, those cheap ones couldn't be THAT far off.

Tick Tock Tick Tock

Yep, it was really there! The smiley face told me it was game on! This was really happening! I was ovulating!

I told Steve, and went to a friend's for lunch. I was tempted to call her to tell her on the drive, I was so excited. Erin had been there for me this entire time and had a one-year-old herself, so she knew how exciting this was that we were trying. I am pretty sure getting to know her daughter, Gemma, was another little seed that made me think about being a mother more than I had before.

Steve and I discussed it later on, celebrating the fact that my body was finally hormonally balanced again. We decided that it was okay to start trying for a family right away; what did we have to lose?

If it worked, we would have a beautiful child to celebrate. Sure, it wasn't the BEST time for his career, but was there ever a good time?

If it didn't happen this month, we could celebrate when my period arrived. I had overcome amenorrhea!

So we did ;)

I know this sounds crazy, but about a week later, I knew I was pregnant.

I am not sure how. I am not sure why. I just knew.

I actually went out to dinner with one of my good friends, Morgan, the evening I first had the feeling, and I told her that. She was excited, but obviously, we both knew it was too early to really take it seriously.

Funny side note: Her response was, *"Well, of course you are. You are just like Kate Middleton who everything just happens perfectly for."*

I laughed, but it turned out she was right, I WAS like Kate Middleton with falling pregnant quickly. I was also like Kate Middleton with how sick I ended up in that first trimester. I ended up cursing Morgan (in a joking way…kind of :p) for comparing me to Kate and making me end up really sick too.

I have always been an intuitive person, and I just knew I was pregnant. I felt different somehow.

Feeling a little different transitioned into a want, no a NEED, for Late July Jalapeno Lime Chips. I could not get enough of them. I was going through bags of them every week, sometimes a bag in a day. I have never been much of a chip fan, and those who know me know that I have never been a lover of spicy or citrus flavored foods, but they were just the best thing in the world.

Pregnancy craving? It has to be, right?

Well, turns out it was.

The wait to find out took FOREVER. I knew it in my heart, but you can never really know until you take that test.

I know lots of other people like to take the test in private, and find a creative way to tell their spouse, but I just felt like this was as much Steve's (potential) baby as mine. We had to do it together.

The earliest day I could take it where it would be accurate (May 28, 2017); I had my pregnancy test waiting, and woke Steve up at 5am to take it. He was barely awake; my mind was already buzzing with what ifs.

We went into the downstairs bathroom, I dipped it in my pee (yep, still no nicer way to do it), and walked out the room. We left it and I paced the kitchen for a few minutes. Steve, being Steve, just chilled as if it was any other day. Probably once again asking himself why he married a crazy person.

We went back in there together, holding hands, and saw the words on the bar: pregnant.

I fell to the floor crying. Steve had tears in his eyes; we cried together and took in this moment. I will never forget that as long as I live. We were gonna be parents!

Just under 8 months later, Bailey Grace Picucci was born into the world. Just over three weeks early, but absolutely perfect in every way.

The day after she was born, I remember looking down at my belly and thinking about how flat it was. Possibly the perspective of having a HUGE belly out in front to having most of it leaving your body within a few hours, but I felt so proud of it. I felt strong and confident; look at what my body had done!

I am never going to take it for granted again.

That feeling stayed with me for a while; I was content with my body, and in awe of how quickly it was able to recover from such an intense change.

Around six weeks after I gave birth, the negative thoughts began to creep in. I had not really lost any more weight since the birth (or it didn't feel like it), and even though I was only 10lbs more than what I weighed when I fell pregnant, I felt frustrated that the 10lbs seemed to make me look different to what I wanted.

I didn't look like the women in the magazines. I hadn't bounced back in 6 weeks. Did that mean I didn't I want it enough?

I had a few photos of me running that I nearly didn't post, because my eyes darted right to my stomach, bulging over my waistband. My size M clothes were still tight. For someone who had been an XS the rest of her life, I struggled to get my head around it. I knew a medium could not be further from huge, and I knew I was being absolutely ridiculous worrying about it, but it was how I felt.

Looking back, and now that I have been in the "normal size" world for a little longer (compared to being underweight), I see that not only do brand sizes vary wildly, but the number or letter really does not mean ANYTHING.

When I was younger, I always wanted to try to fit into the smallest size I could, to be able to say (to no one, because who does that?!) I was a certain size. As you get older, you realize that squeezing yourself into a smaller size doesn't do anyone any favors. NO ONE knows your size, it's not like the label shows on the outside, AND you feel like crap because it is tight and uncomfortable! I wish right after pregnancy (or even before) I had just swallowed my pride and picked up some bigger clothes, yes, even if that meant a large. It would have done so much for my confidence.

Thankfully, I decided to post these photos I wasn't confident about on my social media anyway, just to prove a point. To show others, and more importantly myself, that it didn't matter. No one could tell, and if they could, they were either inspired by me sharing because they too had one of those little extra bellies, OR they were trolls, who really, I didn't care about whatever they thought.

The temptation to diet or to restrict my calories to get back to a weight I was comfortable with began getting harder to ignore. I wasn't going to go crazy and cut back to 1500 calories or anything. I would justify it with, "I just want to lose a little bit." If I lost that weight, I would feel better about myself, right?

Then I thought about the chain reaction it might cause.

That would put me in the exact situation I was in before. Didn't I JUST learn less than a year ago, that being thinner didn't make me happier, that I was HAPPIER after I put on the weight and had a "normal" weight?

What was 10lbs?

NOTHING.

AND I had some very real reminders that were ever-present in my mind. If I did this, I would get into the habit of doing it when I wasn't happy about how I looked, which would ultimately model those behaviors for my daughter. If I fell into the trap of allowing my outer appearance to rule how I felt about myself, Bailey would grow up learning that too. I HAD to snap out of it.

AND if I restricted, I would be taking the calories from her. My body was holding on to that weight for a reason. It needed it. I was so hungry for a reason, and if I took that away from her, maybe I wouldn't be as good at producing milk or looking after her anymore with low energy, and she would struggle to grow appropriately.

All of a sudden, I stopped caring again.

All thoughts about aesthetics and what people would think disappeared. Once again, fueling my body, making sure it was functioning correctly, became the priority. I knew if I wanted to truly overcome amenorrhea, I had to make sure I was eating enough to give my body what it needed to feel safe and calm.

If I feel hungry at all, I eat, even if it has only been a short while since I last ate, or even if I went to bed feeling stuffed, but still woke up ravenous.

It took 11 months for my period to come back after having Bailey. I was still breastfeeding three times per day, but my boobs had returned to a size I was used to, and I noticed she was not taking in as much.

It was such a wonderful feeling knowing I had come full circle. I had officially overcome amenorrhea. I was back to running 70 miles per week, still breastfeeding, I had my period, and best of all, food was no longer something to stress about. That was the biggest difference I noticed. I didn't obsess over what I did or didn't have any more. If I wanted something, I ate it, and there was no guilt or planning about how I would make up for it later; food was only that, food! Something to enjoy, not something to fear.

It wasn't about getting my period back and then slowly bringing my weight back to where it had been, or increasing my running to see if I could play with fire and keep it. Those thoughts were gone. My body was healthy, functioning as it should be, and I intended to keep it that way.

So now, you know my story, in full detail.

Why did it take me nine years to talk about my struggles with amenorrhea? Why did it take me nine years to really do something about it?

You probably already know. The same reason you probably didn't tell your friends and family.

Shame.

We feel shame for not being normal, not being able to function "correctly." Looking back now, I am angry with myself for thinking that, for not being brave enough to share, but also for allowing the fear of being judged to bring that shame. Shame that was not deserved. For allowing my amenorrhea to affect how I viewed myself as a person.

Guilt is something you did that made you feel bad. Shame is feeling like who you ARE is wrong.

No woman with amenorrhea should ever be made to feel ashamed of her body OR who she is; there is nothing to be ashamed of, and hopefully this book will help you see that too.

That being said, it is NOT healthy to be without a menstrual cycle, and as much as doctors try to brush it off by saying, *"just stop running"* (if you even could just give it up like that, but especially when a physician tells you to), that is not the way to go. It might bring it back temporarily, but you have removed something you truly love from your life, while also not solving the problem. For most of us, we would lose it as soon as we started getting back to running again.

Thankfully, the awareness of this issue with female athletes and periods has changed a lot since I first "came out" with my story, and there is more research available, more resources for you to listen to and learn from (that is exactly why I created my Pregnancy and Postpartum Series), and things are moving in a good direction.

That is also why later in this book, you will see that I have shared some insights from Meg Shrier, the Harvard Sports dietitian, who has been to many conferences about this topic in recent years. There is more known about amenorrhea and RED-S, and I think it is only going to continue to become a topic of conversation.

My goal is to be able to say that you have amenorrhea with the same ease you could say that you have an ear infection, and it seems to be headed that way. I am not sure we will ever truly get there, but we can get comfortable saying it around other runners…or at least other female runners.

I know there is a stigma associated with amenorrhea saying that no period=anorexic, which can be hard to accept whether or not you do need help with your relationship with food. It changes the way people look at us, and the judgment from others does not bring about good feelings.

For years, I allowed people to tell me that not eating enough was the only reason I didn't have a cycle. I knew it wasn't that simple, but I just didn't have the knowledge to back it up. There are other factors, and they each have a part to play.

I have had the fortune of getting to know Dr. Rinaldi and Stephanie Buckler who have been very helpful along this process.

So why do WE lose our periods?

This is the question we all want to know. All of us with amenorrhea just want to know one simple thing:

How can some people lose their period at a seemingly normal weight, with low or high volumes of training, and others are able to hold theirs steady no matter how many miles they run or how much they weigh…or how little they eat?

I think it is time I explain a little more about why it happens from what I have learned. Then we can discuss why this happens to us, and why it is not actually as bad as you might think it is. Really!

This book explains all the factors that can cause lack of menstruation, but keep in mind this is just a brief overview. This book is mostly about the moral support for you going through it. There are much better sources on the "why." I am like your emotional coach, but you still need a medical professional, or at least some medical insight to actually do it right.

What are the Causes of Amenorrhea?

Before I get to those, let me just say that this all comes down to how incredibly smart and intuitive our bodies are. I am always telling my superstars that our bodies know best, especially when it comes to running. If we listen to what they are telling us, that is where we can perform at our best at everything we do.

When your body realizes it is in danger for any reason, and that having a baby would not be a good idea as it may not survive the harsh conditions you are living in (primitive, but true), it will shut down your reproductive system to save the energy for your other systems.

Smart. Doesn't make it any less frustrating though, does it?

Most people know about the first two factors that can put your body in that fight or flight mode. Your body senses a scarcity of some kind and views it as dangerous. Many people you probably already have met and will come to meet in your journey will assume these are the only causes of amenorrhea (they are not).

However weight, calories, and exercise definitely play the biggest part, and if you are extreme in any of them, it is almost guaranteed you will not have a period, especially if you are sensitive to it, like I am. That being said, there are three other factors that can increase the likelihood of amenorrhea according to what I read in *No Period. Now What?* and I will go into them after.

Restricted Eating

This is the biggest reason a cessation of periods will occur and continue.

If you are not eating enough to fuel your body, how can you possibly fuel another person to grow as rapidly as they need to to survive inside you and have enough milk to support the baby once it is out?

Your body is saving your future child from what it fears might be a dangerous situation of starvation (even if you are not actually technically starving).

Despite initially being in denial about this one, I eventually had to admit it was part of the problem. After going to see various nutritionists and consultants who told me that I was eating enough and covering all the food groups, I began to believe that this was nothing to do with my amenorrhea, surely it couldn't be? The nutritionists had backed me up on that!

It was only once I started to work with Nancy Clark, a very well-known registered dietitian, that I realized I was not doing as well in this area as I thought, and as much as you might hate me saying this to you, neither are you. We may think we are eating enough, and we can even get other nutrition experts to agree, but this is where a registered dietitian is critical.

We will go into more of what this means later. For now, know that restricting your diet in any way, be it the types of foods you consume, the volume of food you eat, or seeing any food whatsoever as a "bad food" you do not ever allow yourself to have, are all warning signs that this might be an issue for you.

Ready for a hard truth?

If you have ever found yourself thinking, *"How am I hungry again? I can't possibly be hungry now, I had better wait at least x before I allow myself to eat again,"* then you ARE doing this, and you are contributing to your amenorrhea.

Before we go on to the next point, I want to bring up something that will help you understand what is going on here, and what the research is currently discovering. This is something you will see more about in the future, we are just scratching the surface here, but it is important to mention.

After talking to Dr. Meg Steffey Schrier, Sports Dietitian at Harvard for a Running For Real Podcast episode, I realized I needed to include something on RED-S, as it is important for runners of every level to be aware of the consequences, even if they do not have amenorrhea as a symptom.

However, as runners susceptible to amenorrhea, we need to be extra careful. As you will see, an interruption in menstrual cycle is just one of the symptoms.

Let's let Dr. Shrier explain it better:

The term Relative Deficiency in Sport (RED-S) is defined as "impaired physiological function including, but not limited to, metabolic rate, menstrual function, bone health, immunity, protein synthesis, cardiovascular health caused by relative energy deficiency. The cause of this syndrome is energy deficiency relative to the balance between dietary energy intake and energy expenditure required for health and activities of daily living, growth and sporting activities" (Mountjoy, 2014).

But what does this mean?

Bottom line: when you are not consuming enough calories required to meet the needs for your training load you can be considered at RED-S.

Additionally, low energy intake (i.e., your daily calorie intake) and/or increased exercise can cause the balance to lean towards deficiency. For this reason, it is important to make sure you are hitting your nutritional needs to be at an energy balance for sport, so it not only does not affect your metabolic functions but also does not affect your performance.

Another factor to take into consideration is disordered eating, which can also play a part in preventing athletes from hitting their fueling needs for sport. Finding a sports RD who works with either RED-S and/ or disordered eating can aid in hitting energy balance for sport.

RED-S symptoms can range from menstrual irregularity to gastrointestinal problems, as well as decreased immune function. Changes in mood, including irritability and depression, have been noted. Research has shown that changes in estrogen and progesterone levels, even silent ones, can cause negative effect on bone. (Mountjoy, 2014). An effect of menstrual irregularity is the negative change in bone health, which can increase the risk of stress fractures and general injury risk overall.

Finally, there are potential performance effects of RED-S to consider. Research has shown that a person can have a decrease in cardiovascular endurance as well as a decrease in muscular strength. Lastly, athletes can also experience decreased coordination and concentration as a result of deficient caloric intake. It is important that all of these factors are taken into consideration when determining the importance of hitting your daily energy needs for training.

This should make you look differently at all those runners whom you may have envied in the past, wondering how they were able to get away with eating barely anything, and see that by your body not giving you a period, it is protecting you. Your body cannot talk, but it is letting you know that your calories are in a deficiency, and you need to change that quickly. Others are not so lucky. As you can see, menstrual irregularity is just one of the symptoms, but there are many side effects to putting yourself at RED-S, and especially as we think to the future about our return to running or sport, we need to make sure we are getting enough calories in to balance out our activity, even if that does mean eating a lot more than others around you.

As Dr. Schrier states, not only are we at risk of bone issues, but it also will decrease your performance. Nancy Clark also said this to me about potentially running faster had I eaten more when I was working with her during my recovery.

My point with sharing this information from Dr. Schrier is to not only help you recognize that maybe you have been in calorie deficit without realizing it, but to also allow you to be aware of loved ones who may also be at a deficit. You may want to pass on this information to them, if you think they may need to increase their caloric intake. .even if they do not have menstrual irregularity or even if they are not female. RED-S is not limited to females; men are just as likely to be RED-S as women are.

One final thing to note though, just as you may not have listened to comments about yourself being too thin in the past; our loved ones can react badly to us telling them what to do, so tread carefully.

Weight and Weight Loss

This one is also a common assumption. If you are not getting your period, your weight is not high enough. If you lose weight quickly, this may be the reason for the irregularity and cessation of your menstruation.

This again, makes sense.

If your body senses that you do not have enough body fat, you are not going to be able to support a baby.

I only had my body fat percentage measured once…which is a funny story in itself:

I was going to the chiropractor's one day after I finished my run at Dr. Mike's office (as I often did). His office is above a bariatric surgery office, and I was going up the stairs when I heard someone running after me. One of the women from the bariatric surgery asked me if I would be interested in getting my body fat measured. They were curious to see what mine was after they had seen me running in the area many times and knew I was in great health. After working with unhealthy patients every day, they wanted to see what I came up as.

Well, why not? Would be interesting to know, and helpful for them.

So, I had my body fat measured. It came out at 16%. Low, but not crazy low, especially as Steve had told me in the past he had measured 5% once!

And that is how I randomly had my very accurate body fat measurement.

Anyway, back to the point:

Various doctors over the years (including my endocrinologist) told me that my weight was not the cause of my amenorrhea. I had been at various weights during my time with no period, and that did not seem to make a difference.

However, looking back now, I can see that although I was not in an unhealthy weight category, I was technically in the "normal" zone for BMI; it was not high enough for MY body. It links back to the previous section; I was not eating enough for what my body needed, and therefore my weight was lower than it was comfortable being, again sensing starvation as a serious threat.

As frustrating as it is, we have to keep reminding ourselves of this. Others may be able to get away with weighing less, but we are in this special group (and yes, you will learn it is special in a good way) who cannot.

If you have lost more than 10lbs in a short amount of time (within a few months), this could have been what caused your body to retreat the way it did in the first place. Most likely, the weight you were at before that weight loss, or more specifically, where your body was at before you lost your period, is where your body wants to be.

This is a great time to look at your family; what do your mother, sister, aunt, grandmother look like? Are they a lot bigger than you? Maybe your body shape needs to be closer to theirs. If they are overweight, I understand you do not want to put yourself in an unhealthy situation the other direction, for your long-term health, but I am more talking about your shape.

I found once I gained the weight, it wasn't much, but my body shape closely resembled my mother and grandmother. Why? Because that was genetically where my body was predetermined to be.

Ask yourself, is your body fat percentage high enough? Would it do any harm to gain a little weight to see what happens?

Exercise

This is the one that caught me off guard a little when I revealed my secret. I knew it was possible for runners of every level, but I didn't know how big of a problem it was in the general population. You do not have to be an elite runner, a high mileage runner, or even a runner at all to lose your period. It can happen with any type of exercise and even just a combination of high intensity workouts.

How so?

Dr. Nicola Rinaldi, who has spent the ten years since her own amenorrhea recovery researching and helping others to likewise restore their cycles and fertility, can explain it better than I can:

I'm not a runner, but for me it was a combination of restricting my (caloric) intake and playing ice hockey, volleyball, squash, lifting weights, biking, and golf – all of which probably adds up to the same stress on a body – that led to my missing period.
-Dr. Nicola Rinaldi of *No Period. Now What?*

Dr. Rinaldi is the author and researcher of the book, and she thought it would be good to clear up any confusion, so let's dig into this a little deeper. Here is what she found about exercise and amenorrhea.

Exercise and Amenorrhea

When people hear about the idea that running (or other high intensity exercise) can play a part in causing missing periods, a frequent response is to comment that running is not the problem, it's the (under)eating.

This is incredibly difficult to tease apart. People who say, "It's not the running" will point to themselves or others who run at a high level and continue to get regular periods (note – a regular bleed does not always indicate a fully functioning menstrual cycle! (1)). But...on the other hand, for women who do experience amenorrhea, many do not recover missing periods solely by increasing their caloric intake, but only after cutting out high intensity exercise. So—does exercise "cause" amenorrhea? Maybe, maybe not. But, what I can tell you is that for many it likely does play a part either in the initial loss of period, or certainly in preventing recovery.

In fact, it is usually some combination of undereating, exercise, and stress, that cause amenorrhea and *each* of those factors typically needs to be addressed for periods to return.
And it's not just our experience; there is also a large body of medical/scientific literature to back up these ideas. All of this and so much more is included in No Period. Now What?—it's not just about detailing recommendations for recovery; it includes a comprehensive dissection of the science underlying hypothalamic amenorrhea as well as the basis for the recovery recommendations we make.

I am going to distill some of that science here to illustrate how running (or other high intensity exercise) can potentially play a part in causing missing periods—or perhaps it is more accurate to say prevention of period recovery.

Control of the Menstrual Cycle

To explain how exercise might affect periods, and the return of missing periods, we need to start at the beginning, which is the control of the menstrual cycle. Contrary to popular belief that estrogen is the dominant hormone, the cycle in fact begins with gonadotropin releasing hormone (GnRH) release from the hypothalamus, leading to follicle stimulating hormone (FSH) release from the pituitary, which begins the egg growth and maturation process.

The growing egg then releases estrogen as it nears maturation, leading to the release of luteinizing hormone (LH) that triggers ovulation. After ovulation, progesterone is secreted by the collapsed follicle for about two weeks – when this progesterone production stops, your period arrives.

When the hypothalamus is repressed, the GnRH pulses are not sufficient to get that egg maturation process started, and therefore, there is no ovulation and no period.

Exercise and Stress

Running and/or other high intensity exercise have been demonstrated to increase stress hormones like cortisol, cortisol-releasing hormone (CRH), adrenocorticotrpic hormone (ACTH), and b-endorphins.

Cortisol, CRH, and b-endorphins all directly repress the hypothalamus. The repressed hypothalamus no longer secretes gonadotropin-releasing hormone (GnRH) at the rate required for growth and maturation of an egg, which means no ovulation and no period.

These claims are supported by a study performed by Hill et al. (2) where cortisol and ACTH levels were measured in men at varied activities levels: the researchers took a pre-exercise sample, then had the subjects* rest or exercise at 40%, 60%, or 80% of VO2max.

Blood samples were drawn before beginning exercise, then immediately after completion of 30 minutes of exercise. The study was well controlled with subjects (12 exercise-trained men with VO2max > 90% for their age) performing each test separated by a minimum of 48 hours, at the same time of day, and the order of tests was different between subjects.

The results were striking – there was no difference in cortisol levels when exercising at 40% max intensity, but a significant 30% increase at 60% max exercise intensity, and a 62% increase in cortisol at 80% of max exercise intensity.

One interesting observation was there were some people, exercising at 60% VO2max, who did not have much of an increase in cortisol. That is partially why we harp on the idea in No Period. Now What? that every person's situation, path to amenorrhea, and recovery journey, is different.

But, at 80% VO2max, pretty much every subject is experiencing an increase in cortisol.

As far as ACTH goes, results were similar – essentially no change in ACTH upon resting or exercising at 40% of max intensity. At 60% exercise intensity an average 63% increase in ACTH was observed, at 80% max exercise intensity, the increase in ACTH was more than three-fold higher (330%)!

Stress and the Menstrual Cycle

Both of these hormones (as well as other stress-related hormones that are likewise increased by exercise) are sensed by the hypothalamus (3). Then there are also mechanisms by which the stress hormones can suppress the reproductive system at other levels, including the endorphins that we all love from high intensity exercise…while they make us feel good and "less stressed" – in fact, those are also working to suppress our hypothalamus and reproductive system.

These stress hormones affect the neurons in the hypothalamus that produce gonadotropin-releasing hormone (GnRH) that in turn causes the pituitary to release FSH and LH (4).

It is important to note that these effects are not immediate; I don't know anyone who goes for one run and loses her menstrual cycle. It is likely a compounding effect over time, of both the exercise-related stress suppression of the hypothalamus as well as chronic underfueling in many who perform high intensity exercise – sometimes intentional and sometimes not. Our hunger signals often don't account for the calories burned by exercise (5). It also may be that exercise does not play any role in the loss of menstrual cycles, but once your period is missing, that exercise prevents their return. It is common to start work on period recovery by eating more without making changes to exercise routines; few people find this effective.

You are much more likely to regain missing periods by both increasing energy intake (and range of foods) and decreasing or cutting out high intensity exercise.

References are in the resources section.

Phew! Well, there is the science, and Nic was the one who convinced me to go "all in" and texted me back and forth for months after when I would become frustrated.

Going all in isn't always easy, but I am SO glad I did.

Yes, the weight gain.

Yes, the cold turkey stopping of running. I feel in my heart that it was the right thing to do.

As you can probably guess, the exercise component was pretty significant to me, a big reason my body was in fear. It makes sense though, right?

Running 90 miles a week, of course your body is in a state of distress, how would you possibly be able to look after a baby if you are always running from something? Our bodies don't know the sedentary life we live the rest of the time; they just fear we are running from something.

But, the key thing here is the intensity, not even necessarily the miles. If you are sitting here thinking, *"well, I only run xx miles a week, nowhere close to 90, so why am I dealing with this?"*

Actually, from what I have read, the volume of training is really not as important as the intensity. For 14 years of my life, other than maybe 4-6 weeks a year, I had run 2-4 hard workouts per week, in addition to the high volume of miles.

When I started having irregular periods for the very first time, I was actually only running about 30 miles a week, but three of those days were very intense track workouts at Bedford and County Running Club in England.

When I lost it again the second time (and pretty much for good), it was a combination of losing weight and training with more intensity. I believe that especially as I am able to put myself into a deep well, push my body so much harder than it should be capable of in races (and previously in workouts too), it was just too intense for my body.

Are you someone who is able to push themselves hard and dig down deep? Do you often fall into the trap of running harder than you should be? Do you like to run hard?

The authors of *No Period. Now What?* class running as a high intensity exercise.

All of it.

It doesn't matter if you are running easy or hard, it is still very hard on your body. That is why there is such a big correlation between running and irregular periods.

Ask yourself, what is more important to you? Getting that adrenaline rush or thinking about your future health?

Don't worry if it is exercise right now. It was for me for nine years! Not that I recommend ignoring your symptoms, I just mean that I get it. Hopefully this book can help you to change your mind, but either way, do not feel shame for feeling this way. I felt it too.

I know it is frustrating; after all, running is meant to be good for us. All those studies showing how much healthier runners are than the rest of the population.

And then there are all the media messages bombarding us, telling us how we are getting fatter and we NEEEEDDD to exercise.

How are you meant to fight against that by stopping running, gaining weight, and doing nothing?

It's not as easy as it sounds, I can tell you that from experience, I did it. More on that later.

Cutting down or out the exercise that you love can be one of the absolute hardest things you will go through, especially because there will be many people who just don't understand. But the results on the other side – restored fertility and more balance in your life – are so very, very worth the struggle.
- Nicola Rinaldi

When was the last time you took some time off? Do you push your body hard? Has tired become the new normal for you?

Stress

This one is talked about less, but it plays a huge role.

Have you ever heard anyone talking about how they fell pregnant after they adopted or when they had given up trying completely?

Removing stress or pressure can be the reason this happens.

It is the same with our cycles. It can be physical, mental, emotional, or spiritual stress. Our bodies don't really know the difference; all they know is that they are working too hard to be able to sustain a baby at this time. Dr. Trent Stellingwerff talked about this in my podcast interview with him.

I am a high-strung, Type A, competitive worrier, which makes me the prime candidate for high stress levels, and it is not really surprising that my cycles were gone for that reason, at least partially.

I have a sneaking suspicion you might recognize many of those traits within yourself too.

Of all the people who have reached out to me to share their struggle with amenorrhea, I noticed something interesting. Many were not even runners, but stressful events like a divorce, a bad boyfriend, moving, were enough to cause irregular or missed periods, so if those events can do it, surely other things can too.

Ask yourself, is there a lot of pressure and stress in your life? Are you someone who tends to be GO GO GO all the time?

Genetics

Unfortunately, there is not much that any of us can do about this, but it definitely plays a part. My mum also had low estrogen levels and missed periods, which meant I was predisposed to have issues as well.

Even as a teenager, my periods were never heavy, so that should have given an indication that they could be lost easily... but at that time, I didn't know anyone ever stopped having a period until they went into menopause.

Ask your family members, did any of them have issues?

Is Amenorrhea Serious? Can Amenorrhea Lead to Infertility?

This was always one of my fears, and it was the reason that little voice in the back of my mind felt unease whenever doctors would say it was fine.

Of course it's not fine, if my body is so stressed that it doesn't think I could handle being mother to a baby, surely everything is not okay?

It's not, but we convince ourselves it is as we are not doing any real damage…or so we hope!

The longer you let it go on, the longer you are putting your bone health at risk, and there have been some studies that have shown our cardiac health might be at risk without those female hormones. I guess I will find out if there were any long-term effects sometime in the future, but overall, if you are eating well, avoiding illness and do not struggle with injuries, then you are probably okay…

BUT, and this is a big but…

The longer you leave it, the longer you wait, the more damage you are doing to your bone health and mental health.

Do you really want to play around with important parts of what makes you, you?

I didn't think so.

Some good news though:

I always thought the longer I went, the longer it would take to come back, but actually Dr. Nicola Rinaldi found that was not the case.

Phew!

As I proved when I fell pregnant quickly, having amenorrhea does not do any long-term damage to your fertility, but you have to do the work to get to that point. Actually, Dr. Rinaldi found in her research that often women in our situation are MORE likely to fall pregnant quickly. So once you do the work, you may be able to take advantage of those first few cycles.
I like to think of it like one of those inspiring movies where someone ordinary decides to be the brave one to go out there and take the risk; all the others look on in admiration of the brave one who wants to venture into the unknown. I like to think that it is our bodies' way of putting the strongest one forward first.

I also come from a very fertile family, and I realize how fortunate I was to get pregnant on the first try. Although my mum took years to get pregnant, my grandma had ten children, and my sister also fell pregnant on the first try. Truly showing that once you get your body on track, things can happen very quickly...but also showing that genetics still does come into this in many ways. My grandma's child count was proof of that.

Delaying the process might not make you infertile or even make it take longer to get it back, but at some point, you are going to have to face those mental demons that have prevented you from gaining the weight and reducing your exercise in the past. The longer you leave it, the more ingrained those habits will be within you… meaning it will be harder to break them.

The sooner you address it, the sooner you can get on with your life and believe you, yes you my friend, are enough. You always have been.

What Else Could Amenorrhea Impact if Left Untreated?

For me, and for many reading this book, having a baby is the primary goal, but had this book come to me a year before, I would not have been ready for that conversation.

I would, however, have still urged myself to continue making changes and appreciated the support and reassurance along the way.

I would also have wanted to know about the additional ways I was damaging my body by ignoring it, and hoped that someone like me would have told me about them.

Even if you have absolutely no intention to ever have children, there are many reasons to focus on getting over amenorrhea. You know that, you wouldn't be reading this book otherwise.

In many ways, taking this part of your life and making big changes without that physical goal of having a baby in your arms at the end is a lot more difficult than it is for those who do want to get pregnant.

What am I saying?

Well done, my friend; you are being brave, showing your strength and care for your future.

If you go as long as I did without having a period, you know deep down that there are some long-term consequences. They discuss these in _No Period. Now What?_ in a lot more detail, but this includes having serious bone density issues, either now or in your future.

If you haven't had a bone density scan yet, I would suggest getting one, as it can show how serious the impact on your bones has been. If you have been struggling with one injury after the next, especially if it is stress fractures or bone injuries, which are a serious warning flag that you are playing with fire by allowing your amenorrhea to continue. It is difficult to rebuild lost bone, especially once you are older than 30 (and trust me, even if you are much younger, those years will fly by and 30 will be here before you know it!), and you are better preventing damage before it happens.

If you have been on birth control, that might slow the damage, but again, taking that is not really solving the problem, and as we are told not to be on birth control for a long time, even that solution can be short lived.

No Period. Now What? also reported that we could have an increased risk of heart disease, and that women with amenorrhea are at a much higher risk of atherosclerosis (narrowing arteries that go to the heart). Not exactly something we want to consider in the future. If you get your period back now, you can reverse the effects.

I have already talked a lot about the mental distress and frustration we experience knowing that our bodies are not working as they should. We know that our self worth being tied to the way we look is not healthy, and we know we want to be better people.

Even if having a baby is not the goal, I promise you that the peace of mind and the confidence you will get from recovering your cycles will be worth more than you think in every area of your life.

But you already know that, you wouldn't be reading this otherwise.

Baby or not, YOU are important, and YOU deserve love and healing.

Help Me Get My Period Back

So you are ready to do this.

Make the changes you need to make to get your period back. It might take a few weeks; it might take a few years. Your journey is your own, and as much as you don't believe me yet, you WILL be glad this happened, you WILL learn so much about who you are, particularly how STRONG you are as a person. You may end up losing some muscle mass and losing some running memories temporarily, but you will gain so much more.

I am going to break the next few chapters down into layers of recovering your cycle. Where to start and gradually getting more involved and intense. I will start with the "easiest" things to change, and as we move along, I will get to the more drastic changes you may have to make if those do not reveal anything or get things going.

If you are ready to do it all at once as I was, great!

But, that is not the only way, you can do these bit by bit over time, and still get the same result, it just may take longer. Only you will know which approach is going to work better for you.

So let's get to it:

Background Check

As you probably know, if you have done the research I know you have, there are actually two types of amenorrhea: primary and secondary.

Primary amenorrhea is the more serious of the two, and I would strongly recommend going to see a medical professional as soon as possible if you have not ever had a period.

According to WebMD:

Here are some of the main reasons women never get a period:

- Problems with the ovaries
- Problems in the central nervous system (brain and spinal cord) or the pituitary gland (a gland in the brain that makes the hormones involved in menstruation)
- Problems with reproductive organs

As you can see, all of those could turn out to be pretty serious, so if you are beyond age 16, it would be a good idea to get in to see a gynecologist, endocrinologist, or even just your family doctor, who can refer you from there.

I do not have the knowledge to educate you in any way to overcome primary amenorrhea. You can try my suggestions, but I would strongly recommend getting a medical professional to assist you.

This book is mostly about the secondary amenorrhea.

This means that at some point you did have regular periods. Maybe they were a little erratic as a teenager, but for the most part, you did have menstrual cycles as expected at some point in your life.

If this is the case, and you have only recently lost your cycle, chances are a background check will more be for your own peace of mind than anything else. It is always a good place to start, as you would not want to put all your heart and soul into fixing something that no amount of weight gain, rest, and acupuncture is going to change if something fundamental is wrong.

I would suggest starting with your primary care doctor.

To be very honest, most of the primary care doctors I have seen throughout my life have been less than helpful. In fact, for me, they were part of the problem. Asking me the date of my last period upon a checkup for something else like a stomach upset made me feel incredibly awkward, and I felt shame when I responded with, "I do not know."

When that glimmer of hope would arise as they started to ask questions, I would think that maybe, just maybe, this was the person who actually would have something helpful to say.

Except they never did.

Some would essentially shrug their shoulders, clueless as to what to say, writing it off to the exceptional number of miles I ran in a week. In a way they were right, by the point I recognized I had amenorrhea, I was running 60+ miles per week, which IS a lot for anyone to be doing.

The other experts would frustrate me even more.

Nonchalantly, they would say to me, *"well, you just have to stop running."*

I could feel my blood boiling, JUST LIKE THAT!? You just don't get it!?

They didn't.

Why would they?

99% of them were not runners, and most non-runners do not understand runners for many reasons; we are a strange bunch.

The part that angered me was that there was no empathy present, no suggestions for other things to try first. Just that the solution was obvious, and if I was stupid enough to ignore their advice, and then get out of my office, you deserve it.

Okay, maybe not that harsh, but sometimes it sure felt that way.

Despite this, I still think going through them should be the first logical step. Once you voice a concern and have a doctor you trust and like, they should ask you some general questions that can provide clues or at least get you thinking about causes. Important information like whether you are on birth control or what stressful things have been happening in your life lately that could have been a part of the problem, but were hidden in your blind spot.

If they do not ask you questions about your personal history, and seem to be unwilling to consider other factors or help you, go find someone else.

In most situations, the answers you give may baffle them a little, in which case, it is time to move up to the next professional.

If they do not refer you on their own, I would suggest you continue to press for an answer, for a way to fix this problem; they can set you up with some blood tests, and get you referred. Make it seem more urgent, more upsetting if you must (waterworks may help a little :p), if they are not taking it seriously.

For me, the next step was an OB/GYN, and likely, that will be next for you.

This is the professional who will check your internal reproductive organs through an ultrasound. Not the most pleasant experience, most of us know that already, but it is practical, and should be one of the first checks.

There are other health issues that can have similar symptoms to amenorrhea, but this will rule some of them out. OB/GYN practitioners are more likely to have resources of people who might be able to help if they are unsure themselves. If you are looking to become pregnant after you regain your cycle, you can also use the added bonus of getting to know the person who may deliver your child. Are they the right person for you? In my case, my OB/GYN, Dr. Jennifer Fuson, was absolutely the person I wanted!

As frustrating as it is to keep explaining your story over and over again each time you see someone, you go up a little higher in the food chain while specifying in the niche. Your chances of finding a professional who knows more about this area and is not going to judge you with their opinions about running is more likely.

Once you are through the basic background checks on your primary health and your reproductive organs themselves, you will be moved to the next level of assessment.

Blood Work and Further Tests

This could be through an endocrinologist, if you are lucky enough to have been referred there. I would try to be pushy with your doctor to get to see someone like this. They have a lot more experience in this area, and for me, Dr. Wendell Miers was the first person I saw who I felt actually understood me. Not only because he is a runner, but because he seemed to actually understand what was going on with my body itself.

I asked him for a few words on what we are going through from his standpoint; here is what he said:

Hypothalamic amenorrhea is diagnosed once other causes of amenorrhea have been excluded. Workup includes laboratory work and usually an MRI of the pituitary gland. It is caused by low energy availability and stress. The brain recognizes that there isn't enough energy stored to sustain a pregnancy and thus ovulation stops. The female hormone levels often return to prepubertal levels. The treatment is relatively straightforward. It entails restoring positive caloric balance and gaining weight. Usually the percent body fat needs to increase enough to restore the hormonal function and ovulation. -Dr. Wendell Miers

If you do not see an endocrinologist, this may be getting your blood work done through a service like Inside Tracker (use code TINAMUIR for 10% off), back through your family doctor, or if you are really lucky, a reproductive endocrinologist. I did not see someone for this, but from what I hear, this is the gold standard.

Just a note, they will probably take many vials. I remember having 13 taken at one point! I saw it as the more the better; the more they take, the more assessments that could potentially give you an answer.

Your blood work will come back, and they will explain to you where everything fits within the ranges of normal. Cortisol levels (which indicate your level of stress), your iron level, and the many various hormones within the blood are all going to show a little part of the puzzle.

Don't take too much notice of the hormone levels themselves in terms of where they are within the normal ranges. Mine tended to fall within the normal range most of the time, and these numbers are supposed to fluctuate within a month, but I found mine did not vary too much between visits.

As tempting as it is, try not to read too much into this yourself; leave it to the professionals, they are the ones who have been trained to do so.

If you are not satisfied with the results of the blood work and it did not give you anything at all, that could be causing your amenorrhea; you can also go for a urine analysis or DUTCH test. For me, this didn't really shed any light on anything new, but it is more accurate for measuring your reproductive hormones, and as you measure multiple times within a day, it can give indicators that are more accurate.

Word of warning though, these can be expensive. If you are very much into the natural, homeopathic method, you might be prepared to pay for it, but full disclosure, I was given an assessment for free through *Nourish Balance Thrive*.

Medication

I mentioned in my story that I was put on some hormones to try to kick start my cycles again, and from speaking to others, this is a common approach. One that makes sense in theory, right?

If your body has rather lost its way, you are giving it a little reminder of what it is supposed to be doing every month.

Except, as I mentioned for myself and many others, it usually doesn't work, because there is something deeper going on. Worse still, medication such as birth control can mask the symptoms, giving some kind of bleeding each month, which makes it seem like all is well, when in fact, you are not ovulating. Remember I shared about Esther earlier in the book?

Looking back now, I am not even sure it was the right thing to do to force my body to have that period all those years ago.

Sure, it proved a point that I COULD menstruate, but I already knew that. I had a period as a teenager. Instead, that allowed me to put the blinders on and accept that I just wasn't going to have cycles, rather than figuring out what was going on.

Before that forced bleeding, had I continued to take steps to figure out WHY I was not having a period, maybe I could have avoided having to take such a drastic step later (or put my long term health at risk!).

I know it can be tempting to jump on the hormone control train, and by all means, try the progesterone challenge, but don't get your hopes up. If it works, great, maybe your body was just a little out of whack; just take it as a warning that your body is sensitive and you need to give it extra care (and calories) to make sure you are able to keep your cycles.

If it doesn't work, though, take that as the huge red flag that it is, and dig deeper to find out what is going on…and not just through more medication!!

If you are trying to overcome amenorrhea in order to get pregnant, this becomes even more important. Many medical professionals will be quick to jump on the ovulation stimulator medication like Clomid (or something similar) route. I have heard of physicians recommending IVF before even trying to fix the things we talked about above, absolutely shocking!

I would be sure to do a lot of research on this. My mum was actually put on Clomid to have me, but she was on it for two years (I don't think they let you stay on it that long anymore). After doing my own research and reading about it in _No Period. Now What?_, I was absolutely adamant I was not going to be put on Clomid or anything else unless it was absolutely necessary and we had tried everything else (except IVF).

I am not saying there is anything wrong if that is your choice, but I would strongly recommend on reading up on it first and giving what I talked about in this book a try before you do. It is not my area of expertise, but it often doesn't solve the problem, and if you don't address your issues now, you might end up addressing them after pregnancy, when you have a lot more hormones and other things going on with your body and mind.

Here is what Dr. Nicola Rinaldi said about this. She is the one who has done all the research and found countless women who have been put on hormones, and then eventually have been encouraged or even pushed towards IVF rather than giving their body a chance to heal itself:

Many medical doctors see very few cases of hypothalamic amenorrhea and don't really understand either the causes or the repercussions. Birth control pills are often prescribed as a Band-Aid, but their 'protection of bones' is debatable, and they're certainly not going to help with getting pregnant. The best long-term solution is to recover your own natural menstrual cycles! -Nicola Rinaldi

Again, I would strongly recommend _No Period. Now What?_ if you want to learn more about this issue; she has a whole chapter on oral medications.

Seeing a Naturopath

As I mentioned in my story, a few weeks before I stopped running I went to see a naturopath. My aunt had been going to see Natasha for years, visiting her one to two times a year, every year, and believing, genuinely believing, that she was working miracles with her health.

My aunt and I are very close; in fact, she and I share values on many different topics, including the law of attraction (universal intelligence), which is met with many raised eyebrows.

However, going to see a naturopath was a little out there, even for me.

My aunt would always come back from her appointment with a huge collection of drops to put in filtered water to help clear up viruses or other things going on in her body. These drops cost a good amount of money (a few hundred dollars); in addition to the cost of the appointment (which wasn't cheap), it made me very skeptical.

However, I was tempted. I had tried everything else, I am very much about holistic health over just taking medication to fix things, and really, other than a few hours of my day and a few hundred dollars, did I really have THAT much to lose? Maybe she would find the answer?

She found me to be in very good health (surprise, surprise!), but did give me some drops to see if we could get my period to come back.

I ended up stopping running within a few weeks anyway, so for me, I will never really know whether the drops had any kind of effect or not. As for recommendations, if you are at the end of your rope, frustrated with the medical industry and prepared to go into it with an open mind, I think going to see a naturopath is worthwhile. Even though it was expensive, for me it was worth it, even just as verification that I was doing the right things to have health as a priority.

They may be a little out there, but if you are a believer in holistic medicine like I am, and you can afford it, might be worth a try. If you do go down this route, just be sure you find someone who has good reviews (I would go by word of mouth rather than through the internet). Natasha is a member of the Alliance of Registered Homeopaths and has an internationally recognized diploma in Complementary Medicine working alongside Orthodox Medicine. Look into those qualifications for someone in your area.

One final thing to mention though, while the treatments a naturopath offers can be helpful, they are unlikely to work without also increasing your fuel and reducing high intensity exercise.

Change the Quality of Your Diet

The next step is to work on something you can change without really altering your life before doing something more drastic. Of all the steps I am going to talk about, this might be the one you find easiest.

I am not talking about gaining weight yet, but more making sure you are getting the right quality of foods.

Our bodies need enough nutritionally dense foods to function correctly. You may find that if you have been neglecting these, just adding them back in is enough to get everything going again.

This would include making sure you have enough healthy fats in your diet.

We went many years thinking fat was scary, it was the thing MAKING us fat, right?

Wrong. Fat is actually very good for you and when you have amenorrhea, it becomes critical to begin your recovery journey. You want to make sure you have enough of it for your body to function correctly. Some of the high fat foods I enjoy are:

- Salmon (and other oily fish).
- Nuts (almonds, cashews, Brazil nuts, hazelnuts).
- Nut butters (I love to make my own almond butter, but regular peanut butter works too).
- Coconut (I love coconut butter by the spoonful).
- Grass fed butter (on everything, especially when you are cooking, use a lot! I love Kerrygold and you can find it at Costco for pretty cheap).
- Grass fed-grass finished (this is important, "grass fed" alone has lost a lot of its meaning in recent years) beef, lamb, pork.
- Free-range chicken thighs.

- Eggs (I love to find a local farm and pick up eggs from them instead of the store; the yolks are BRIGHT yellow, so you know the chickens' diet was good).
- Whole milk (again, I love to use a local farm).
- Cheese (I love strong, sharp cheddar).
- Whole milk yogurt (I actually prefer plain, just add some fruit or something sweeter with it).

There are a lot more, but those are the ones I found easiest to add into my diet.

Try to increase your fat intake to around 30-40% of the foods you consume...but don't get obsessed counting it, just make a rough guess. At this point, the more the better! If you end up eating more calories overall, great! That is not going to do any harm; those are all good quality foods that your body is going to thrive on! If you do put on weight while adding these extra fats into your diet, it is because your body needed them, and that is a good thing!

Now although organic products are ideal, if you are unable to find or afford these foods, conventional fruits, vegetables and meats are better than processed versions of organic that might not even be organic at all. Just try to do your best. It doesn't have to be perfect; I still end up eating out a lot, and I am pretty sure most of the restaurants we go to are not going to always have organic products.

Calcium is another area that is often neglected, and for those of us missing those vital hormones every month, which is slowly harming our bones, calcium becomes absolutely critical.

Be sure to be drinking full fat milk, whole milk yogurts, and eliminate anything that is reduced fat, rather than the full fat kind. That way you're killing two birds with one stone; getting your fats in while consuming the calcium in the dairy.

Take a Few Weeks Off

If you are reading this right now, chances are you are a type A perfectionist, who is able to stick to her schedule, pick goals and go get them.

It has probably been a while since you took a break. Like a real break. Not a few days of easy running, not cross training while you took a week off running after a race, but a good two weeks of complete and total rest.

"But I don't want to lose the fitness I have worked so hard for," you are thinking.

I know, I know. You HAVE worked hard for it.

Look at it this way:

Your body also has worked hard, very hard over the years, so it deserves a rest. Your amenorrhea is proof that it is feeling a little strained, pulled in a few too many directions, and it does not feel like it is able to keep everything working as it should.

You might not be ready to take the full cutout approach like I did, but a few weeks of total rest (WITHOUT restricting your caloric intake) really could be just what you need to kick start your periods to start again.

A few weeks will absolutely fly by, and I am willing to bet that when the 14th day arrives, you will think to yourself, *"Well, that wasn't that bad."*

Maybe part of you will even kinda wish you had a few more days as you were starting to enjoy the extra time… which of course you filled with other things very quickly. In which case, go for it!

The more time you take, the quicker your cycles will return.

A few weeks off running could be just what your body needs, and really, you are barely going to lose anything in a few weeks. At minimum you come out feeling refreshed, and best case scenario (although do not expect it!), you could come out with a period!

Isn't it worth a try?

What would you tell a best friend who came up to you and said she was going to have to take a few weeks off because of an injury, life, or travel after years of being consistent? Would you say, *"What the hell is wrong with you? You are so lazy, get back out there and find the time!"*

No way.

You would reassure her and tell her that she will be fine. You would tell ~~them~~ her a few weeks is nothing and to go enjoy herself. Fitness will be back in no time.

Can you not grant yourself the same well wishes?

Cutting Back on Training

Take a few weeks off with no such luck?

Don't feel bad, very few people are able to get their periods back that quickly and with just a few weeks.

I know, you thought you were going to be one of the lucky ones. You had convinced yourself that was all you needed, and now you feel totally disheartened.

I get it, I thought so too, but I too was wrong. Doesn't mean you are a failure in any way though, just means we have some work to do, together.

Also means you didn't waste your money purchasing this book ;)

So now, it is time for the next step. You are not quite ready to pull the trigger and stop running, but you know you do have to make some changes, and you are ready (not happy though) to do that.

I was at a point with my running where I could give it up. I had become disenchanted with it, and after 14 years of training, I welcomed a break from it.

I understand though, that maybe you aren't at that point. One of the things I am most proud about with sharing my story is that people like you are not waiting until you are in dire need of a change, until you will try ANYTHING to get it to work.

That is a good thing, catching it before it is too late.

I honestly believe if I had not stopped when I did and had continued on to do the Gold Coast Marathon as planned, I would have destroyed my relationship with running forever.

I am not sure I could have ever got back into running again. EVER.

When medical professionals had told me over the years to stop running, they made it seem so simple.

"Just stop."

Yeah, just like that. Whatever. Let me remove my right arm for you while I am at it!

I would become frustrated with them. They didn't understand what running meant to me, they didn't get it because they weren't runners themselves, you can't just stop when you love it so much. Is it worth giving up something you love just for the sake of bleeding, that no one really enjoys anyway?

We all know the answer deep down should be yes, but in reality, it's just not how we feel. Our emotional health is just as important as our physical health, especially when you know it is not affecting your long-term fertility. Nor is the damage going to be drastically changed by waiting a few months to see if maybe you do reach a point where you feel comfortable with stepping away from running.

I get it.

When I was in college and doctors would suggest I stop running to get my cycle back, I had to try not to laugh in their face… or punch them in the face! How could they suggest that? Especially as I was on a full ride scholarship to run in the US. Stop running? Well, then I also give up my degree and go home.

That wasn't going to happen.

As you know, I did reach a stopping point where I could do it, but if you can't, that is not the end of the world.

Now, I am just an experiment of one. I do not have research behind this, and once again, I recommend reading *No Period. Now What?* if you want to know why it is necessary to stop running.

All I am going to say is that from what I have learned through speaking to others, and looking back on what I did, I believe it is possible to resume your cycle without giving up running.

BUT

You knew that was coming, didn't you.

I think the not running aspect is less important than the significant increase in calories (and likely weight gain). If you are prepared to put on weight and run less, you may well be able to resume your cycle. It will take longer, but if you are okay with that, by all means try it.

If you do want to continue running, the gaining weight aspect becomes even more important, and the time it will take to recover becomes longer. You have to decide what is more important to you.

Running or time?

The other part of continuing to run as you overcome amenorrhea is that you have to chop it down, significantly.

If your body is in a place where it is crying out for help, it needs to feel reassured, and the best way to do that is to remove high intensity (and remember ALL running is considered high intensity).

Let's take this a little deeper again for a moment:

As human beings on this earth, we have one real job. Sure, we have plenty of other things that bring us fulfillment and joy, but at the end of the day, we are here to survive, to pass our genes on to the next generation, to keep the population of human beings alive. The reproductive cycle is how that happens.

Each time an egg is released once a month, you have another opportunity to produce offspring. In the past (way, way back), when we were living in caves and our threats were not a damaged egos from someone making a comment on social media, but real threats to our very existence, why would you NOT menstruate?

Because it is not safe to do so. Because you are literally running away from dangerous predators or circumstances. A pregnant woman or a woman with a baby would slow your tribe down; make it vulnerable and unlikely to survive.

The dangers of an animal chasing us may have gone, but not enough time has passed to let our bodies know that we are no longer in danger. The fact that we are RUNNING so hard (and so much), gives it the same fear factor that this is happening again, which will make the reproductive system shut down. It is not safe to have a baby right now.

Most of us who are in this situation are people who can push hard, edge close to our limits and give it our very best. We are the people who will carry 12 bags in each hand, straining our muscles and cutting our fingers, just to make sure we only take one trip from the car to the kitchen. We also struggle to take it slow, in every area of life, but particularly in our running or exercise. We thrive on the challenge of seeing what we are made of.

I get that maybe you are not at the stage where you can step away from running completely, but if you do truly love to run for what it is and you can't imagine a life without it, your alternative is to run short and run easy: **only** easy.

For most of us runners, our bodies are so used to running, easy runs could be classed as low intensity, easy enough to allow your body to settle down.

If you are going to do this without stopping running, you will need to cut out all hard workouts, as in anything that is harder than a jog, AND you are going to have to reduce your volume by half (if not more).

I mean taking it so slow that you can breathe in and out through your nose **the entire time** (yes, even going uphill). The best way to ensure you do keep it easy enough is to use a heart rate monitor to ensure your heart rate stays in the MAF zone, along with cutting your mileage in half to allow your body to calm down.

What is MAF pace you ask?

Maximum Aerobic Function. According to Phil Maffetone himself, use this 180 formula to figure yours out:

To find your maximum aerobic training heart rate, there are two important steps.
1. *Subtract your age from 180.*
2. *Modify this number by selecting among the following categories the one that best matches your fitness and health profile:*

a) If you have or are recovering from a major illness (heart disease, any operation or hospital stay, etc.) or are on any regular medication, subtract an additional 10.

b) If you are injured, have regressed in training or competition, get more than two colds or bouts of flu per year, have allergies or asthma, or if you have been inconsistent or are just getting back into training, subtract an additional 5.

c) If you have been training consistently (at least four times weekly) for up to two years without any of the problems in (a) and (b), keep the number (180–age) the same.

d) If you have been training for more than two years without any of the problems in (a) and (b), and have made progress in competition without injury, add 5.

For example, if you are 30 years old and fit into category (b), you get the following: 180–30=150. Then 150–5=145 beats per minute (bpm).

In this example, 145 must be the highest heart rate for all training

A warning to you as you begin running at MAF heart rate.

It is going to be difficult to run like this. Not in the sense of pushing yourself, but it is going to seem incredibly slow and maybe make you question why you are even bothering at all.

In many ways, that is kind of the point. Just how much do you love to run?

Enough to run very slow?

You **must** stick to this, and maybe it will even help you reach a point where you would rather not be running than running this slow. However, if you want any hope of getting your cycle back while still running, this is your best shot.

I would strongly recommend having your heart rate monitor beep at you if you go above your max heart rate training number, and of course, listen to it! Slow down if it does beep!

If you are prepared to do this and limit your mileage (think first time runner kind of mileage) along with keeping it all very easy, you have a shot. I am not promising anything, but I do know people who have seen it happen.

That being said, remember this way of overcoming amenorrhea will take longer.

If you are impatient, this is probably not the best method for you. Most of the runners I know who have done this have taken at least a year to get their cycles back.

So at the end of the day, do you have to stop running?

No, but you have to ask yourself if you are prepared to wait, remove all intensity, and drastically reduce pace.

You will still need to gain weight, and eat even more calories to make up for the calories you are burning in exercise, but it can be done. Listen to my podcast episode with Tawnee Gibson for more about that one.

This is the route she went down and it worked, but it took a few years, rather than the few months it took me. She also had to overcome an eating disorder and was very honest about her struggle with that. If you are struggling with what you think might be an eating disorder, Tawnee's episode will be especially powerful for you along with the Meg Steffey Schrier and Jessi Haggerty episodes.

Only you can decide if you are prepared to dive in, do everything you can in one go, rip the Band Aid off and go for it, or slowly back away.

I am not saying one is right and one is wrong, but only you can decide which is best for you and where you are.

If you are okay with those, by all means try it.

If that doesn't sound fun to you and defeats the purpose, then maybe you are almost ready for the full cutout stage. For me, I always felt that I would rather not run at all for a few months than run just a little for longer.

Only you can decide if running easy and short is enough for you.

Increasing Caloric Intake

Ready for the hard part? The part you hoped I just never brought up?

Okay, so you have tried altering your diet and nothing seems to have changed. You have taken a few weeks off to no avail. You have backed off your running. Nothing.

That was the situation for me. I tried changing my diet two years before I stopped running and I had taken a few sets of 1-2 weeks off completely, hoping it would be enough. Nope.

When I heard not eating enough fats was one reason a lot of women did not get their cycles, I went all in with the fats. I ate high fat, high protein, low carb. I was going crazy with fats, consuming all I could in the day, hoping it would work.

Of course, it didn't, and I was left with the only other alternative, and maybe you are at that point too. It is time to do what is scary and you hoped it wouldn't come to:

Allowing yourself to eat more, a lot more, especially if you are still running.

Sounds fun for people looking in from the outside, but you probably already know that it is not as fun as it sounds. Because you know that it probably means weight gain, the one thing you want to avoid. As much as you want your cycle to return, you don't want to end up "fat," you fear that once you start binging on these foods, you won't be able to stop eating.

We are told day after day about how addicting sugar is, how the size of your stomach increases as you eat more.

How the heck am I ever going to stop if I allow myself to eat as much as I want of those foods now?

Besides, everyone else is trying to lose weight, trying to be healthier, that just feels wrong that I am allowing myself to eat whatever junk I want when every ad on the radio, TV commercial and more is making me feel guilty for eating, like I am a lazy slob.

I hear you, I felt it too.

There is also a fun side to it, which we need to focus on.

All those foods you have wanted to eat for years, you now get to enjoy and eat them as much as you want. Yes, you will eventually calm it down and get back to a more normal way of eating, but for now, you can have fun with it.

In *No Period. Now What?* they explained that most women with amenorrhea need to get to a BMI of 22-25, which is known as the "fertile zone." As I mentioned, I am not a fan of using weight, but this puts it into context, as most of us have a rough idea of what our BMI is. Before I stopped training as an elite, I was around 19 BMI, which meant I would need to get to around 130lbs to be within the 22-25 BMI range.

Many "fertility foods," which meant lots of ice cream, "junk" food, and…well, whatever the heck I wanted!

Coincidentally, I have been told by a few experts that you should try to make your life resemble what it was like when you last had a regular cycle, which for me would mean back to my time in California, where my weight probably was around my "fertile weight," and my training was very…let's just say…relaxed. ;)

I did end up getting my period back when I hit that exact weight. I believe I was just over 130lbs when I fell pregnant with Bailey, and my body shape pretty closely resembled what it was when I was in California.

There was one major difference though, one thing that really put it into perspective for me:

For years, I had fought aggressively against anyone who told me it was because of a caloric deficit.

In fact, in many of my blog posts, including the one where I announced to the world that I was stopping running, I talked about how I had been assessed by many nutritionists and experts. I had given my food log to probably 10 different people over the years. They all came to the same conclusion: I was doing a good job, getting enough.

And enough it was…to get by, but not enough for my body to feel safe and to function fully.

I don't mind admitting I was wrong, and in this situation, I was.

I was underfueled. Maybe it wasn't by much, but it was for sure a factor.

As I mentioned earlier, Nancy Clark was the one who finally made me realize I was under fueled. As we talked, and I was totally transparent with her, I got that feeling we all hate. In the pit of your stomach. I felt that sinking feeling when it dawned on me that all along I had been wrong. And if you are anything like me, you haaaatttee the idea that the answer was there all along.

I started working with Nancy after I had taken off about 6 weeks of running, not long before I ovulated actually.

I know I could have started menstruating without working with Nancy; it wasn't as if she clicked a button and I was suddenly functioning again.

But, here's the thing:

My mindset towards food and eating would not have changed. I was gaining the weight to get pregnant and had already decided I was going to do whatever it took to get there, but I know myself, and once I did get back into running again, once the training started to ramp up, I would want to lose the weight and would fall back into the same habits again.

Which would only lead to one thing: amenorrhea again and those thoughts telling me that my self-worth as a runner was tied to how much I weighed or how I looked in my running shorts.

I wouldn't have accepted that I was underfueling, and although I would have proved that I could have a period, I could get pregnant, I would not have faced the truth and the demons inside. Therefore, I would still have that underlying unsettled feeling that something wasn't quite right.

Nancy helped me to see that in fact I wasn't eating enough the entire time I was an elite runner, and not just that, she even believed I could have run FASTER had I been fueling better, had I taken in more calories, even if that meant a higher weight to go with it.

I know you have done everything in your power to be the best runner you can be, done the little things to shave time off here and there, but think about that for a moment; what if you have actually been sabotaging yourself all along?

What if YOU could have been FASTER too?

Maybe that would have meant a BQ. Maybe that would have meant you dipped under a major barrier.

That doesn't mean you can't do it in the future, and that is what I am reminding myself of right now. With this new mindset, a body that is fueled, and the right attitude, maybe I can run faster than I did before, a LOT faster, and that is exciting for the future.

It still means you have to do the work now. You have to be prepared to admit you are the reason you are in this situation, intentionally or not; your body is not happy with you, and a professional who is not so emotionally involved is probably the one who will make you see that.

I know seeing a registered dietitian costs money, money you probably do not have, but really, think about it, if you get your mind in the right place, where you can actually look at food as something to enjoy, something to appreciate, how good will that feel! Without that guilt you feel around food, without those calculations as to what you can and can't eat today, it will give you freedom that is worth 1000 times the cost of seeing an RD.

Trust me, I know.

But there is a silver lining here:

Nutrition services generally are covered by health insurance in the US these days. You just need to call your health insurance company to confirm that the insurance policy covers nutrition services (Z71.3 is one billing code that can be used). That takes away the barrier of money in many cases. Worldwide, you may be able to climb your way up the health care chain to get to a dietitian without paying.

Besides, you probably only need a few sessions. I think I have had maybe four sessions with Nancy TOTAL, and the final one was post pregnancy and a quick call, just to make sure I wasn't slipping back into bad behaviors.

Even if you do have to pay, think about it this way:

We are not very good at spending money on ourselves, not on the things that truly matter like this. We would much rather purchase something physical, like a new pair of running shoes or those cute running tights your favorite pro runner is raving about, but at this point in your life, you need to invest in yourself, in WHO you are, not what you look like or what you think you need to impress on social media. Invest in the person you are, becoming the best person you can be.

A registered dietitian was the one person, above all other things, that was the key to changing the way I felt about myself. If you spend money on one thing to overcome your amenorrhea, make it be that. If you get your nutrition right and your mind in the right place around food, the rest becomes a whole lot easier. I promise.

At the time, I was not running at all, and not really exercising either. Nancy calculated that I needed about 2400 calories in the day. Yep, you read that right, 2400 calories without any exercise.

She told me it was best to break it up into buckets. I was to eat 600 calories every four hours. 600 x 4 = 2400. If you are still running, it is going to be significantly more.

To someone who knew calories and how quickly they added up, 2400 really didn't seem like that much to me. I know for some runners, maybe you are one of them, 2400 is probably all they consume even on high mileage days, so that may seem like a lot, but to me, it seemed like a piece of cake (no pun intended!).

I had already been through the bingeing stage the past 6 weeks, eating everything and anything in sight, so I knew I was eaassssillyy surpassing that number of calories and had gotten used to the idea of a lot more coming in than going out.

This next stage in my recovery was about finding a good balance, a place where my body was getting what it needed to recover and heal, without bingeing on ice cream and cake.

HOWEVER, Nancy (and I think you will find most RDs) are NOT about restriction, in any form. If I wanted fried chicken, go have the fried chicken. If I wanted cake with ice cream AND sweets AND frosting, go for it.

That might not be what you expect to hear from an RD, but essentially, if you want that and you have it, you kind of get it out of your system. Eat what you crave and you will feel content.

I had been following my cravings for weeks and I had already gained about 15lbs, so I was ready to get some nutrition back into my diet.

Breaking down 2400 calories into 600-calorie "buckets" every 4 hours immediately sent my mind to one place: dinnertime. Eating just 600 calories at dinnertime seemed like nothing. I had calculated in the past that on average, in the evenings I had consumed about 1000 calories, sometimes more for dinner and dessert, 600 was surely not going to be enough?

Then you look at the start of the day.

At this time, I was waking up at 6am, which meant I needed 600 calories at 6am. Surprisingly hard to do. If you take something like oatmeal, and you have one cup uncooked (which is about 2 cups cooked), that gets you to about 300, HALF of what you need. You tack on some peanut butter, chia seeds, flax seeds, and syrup, have orange juice, and you reach 600.

Phew.

After all that, I was left feeling pretty full. I don't know about you, but unless I go out, I don't think I would ever get that many calories for breakfast, especially not at 6am. If I was going to have a huge breakfast, it would usually be more of a brunch, where I have had some time to build up to it.

While writing this book, Nancy informed me that a "food bucket" can be divided into two meals. The word bucket means the calories need to be consumed within 4 hours. So, you could have 300 calories at 6:00am and another 300 calories at 8:00am.

Anyway, back to my story:

Down goes breakfast, and you get on with your morning. I noticed I wasn't thinking about eating again; I didn't reach for any snacks or think about food in any way. Before I knew it, it was 10am, and guess what, time for another 600 calories. I found I was not really that hungry by this point, but I had committed to it, and so I found a way to get another 600 in. Either another breakfast, or an early lunch.

Soon enough 2pm rolls around, and it is time once again for another meal. By now, I was definitely full of energy, but also very full of food! Again, embracing the opportunity to eat more, I had another 600 calories.

By 6pm, it is time for the final meal of the day, and I had not had a single snack; I just didn't need it with all those meals. Usually I am a big grazer, but not eating this way.

Here is where it gets really interesting though:

I wasn't that hungry for dinner.

I ate what I would consider a normal sized portion of food. No, not what they serve in chain restaurants that are really enough food for a family of four, but a regular serving size, what the American Heart Association or Center for Disease Control recommends, and then I was full.

I felt this way every day that I did as Nancy asked, hungry, but just enough to eat one more normal meal. Sometimes, I would have enough room for a small dessert, but most days, I just felt...full.

Then something really interesting happened:

I just wasn't as interested in dessert anymore. I wouldn't have my handful of M&Ms here and mini Snickers there, and in the evening, I was satisfied with a few squares of dark chocolate or again, a normal size portion of dessert (as opposed to my GIANT size dessert of before). If I baked cookies, I had one cookie. If I had ice cream, I had one serving. If I didn't even have any dessert, I didn't mind that either.

I couldn't believe it!

Me! Someone whose blog was originally named *Insatiable Sweet Tooth* to document my insane sugary creations.

Me! Who could NOT go to bed without having a dessert, even if that meant going out at 9pm looking for a candy bar!

Me! Who would have a giant slice of pie with ice cream for dessert, but would still go straight out to the kitchen after to get some candy, as I wasn't quite satisfied.

Suddenly, the sweet cravings were not there. I still enjoyed eating sweet foods, don't get me wrong, but I wasn't thinking about the next "fix" all the time.

I told Nancy I did actually really enjoy my desserts; they made me happy. How was I supposed to work around that if I didn't want them in the evenings, I didn't have room for them?

She suggested I have my dessert as one of my "meals" early in the day. So I would. Steve and I would go for ice cream at 2pm, or I would have a cookie with something else to get to the caloric recommendation for that "bucket." I would enjoy my sweets throughout my other meals. This is where the fun part comes in; you get to eat foods you really enjoy, but also make new memories while you do it.

In my head, I thought dietitians would tell me sweets are bad and I should limit myself to one square of chocolate a day (yeah, right! Who does that, I certainly don't!), but she didn't. Nancy encourages you to be "curious," and go for what you want.

With one caveat though. You have to actually enjoy it.

No more breezing by the candy dish grabbing something, shoving it in while you're doing something else, and then having another a few minutes later.

Honestly, I am still a little guilty of this.

If you are going to have something that is not nutritionally dense, you had better enjoy it; sit down and appreciate it. If you don't have time now, save it for later.

I feel like that helps, as a lot of the time I wanted that "fix" of sugar, but it wasn't really hitting the spot as I was multitasking, and before I knew it, it was just devoured without really enjoying it.

Just a Little Extra

Without a photographic memory, I cannot remember exactly what I said to Nancy, and what our conversations ended up being about, but I do, however, have my follow up emails. Here are some questions I had for her that you may also be wondering about, and what her responses were.

Tina: Is it a good idea to journal what I am eating?

Nancy: If it helps you learn, yes. If it's a meaningless chore, no.

T: How should I plan if I have a meal out with friends, I am thinking more about lunch than dinner. If I met friends at like 12pm, should I just put off that first meal until 8am?

N: If you have breakfast at 6:00 or 7:00, you will be hungry by 10:00 or 11:00, so you might want to have part of your lunch early—and then at lunch, you might end up having your first and second lunches at the same time. That is, if you eat a bigger-than usual lunch, you won't be hungry for lunch 2.

Hunger is a simple request for fuel. You want to honor that request, and not abuse your body. The goal is to offer your body fuel when it needs it. That is, if you were babysitting and the little baby was crying at 11:00 because it was hungry, would you say "Shut up. You cannot eat until noon."? Doubtful.

Love that way of thinking, so true isn't it!

After each session, my homework was to learn from each day; here is what Nancy suggests we do:

- *At the end of the day, ask yourself:*
  - *What went right?*
  - *What went wrong?*
  - *How could I have eaten better or differently?*
  - *What will I do the next time?*

- *Keep being curious: "I wonder what will happen if I*
  - *Eat candy?*
  - *Have a big dinner?*
  - *Skip a meal?*

By learning from each day, you will learn how to handle every eating experience, be it a restaurant meal, a social event, Thanksgiving, etc.

The more you can trust you can handle different food situations (without "getting fat"), the happier you will be.

You may or may not end up working with Nancy Clark, but I hope this chapter has shown you the importance of working with a registered dietitian over a nutritionist. You can get nutritionist certifications without the intensity of a degree the

RD would have gone to school for, and technically, anyone can call themselves a nutritionist. I took a nutrition class in college, so I could claim that too.

Choosing someone with the RD word next to their name means you are safely choosing someone who is going to know how to help you eat well to fuel your body.

If you go to the website for the Sports and Cardiovascular Nutrition Dietary Practice Group of the Academy of Nutrition and Dietetics., you can scroll the homepage to "Find a SCAN RD," where you can use the referral network to find a local sports dietitian, preferably one who is a CSSD—an RD who is a (board) Certified Specialist in Sports Dietetics.

Hopefully, you are getting this earlier in your amenorrhea journey. Working with an RD would be the first step I would recommend on your journey. I would also recommend working with your primary care doctor, to keep them in the loop on what you are doing. That way, they can keep an eye on your cholesterol and overall health, to make sure you are not putting your body in any danger with this somewhat extreme way of eating.

I would also strongly recommend listening to my podcast episodes with Nancy and Renee McGregor, as well as the eating disorder special with Meg Steffey Schrier and Jessi Haggerty. Nancy's episode is a more general overview of how to eat the right amount for YOUR body, Renee's episode focuses more on Orthorexia (an obsession with healthy eating), and the Meg and Jessi episode covers RED-S and eating disorders. All three are very powerful drivers to change and may make you realize what you have been afraid to admit to yourself.

If You Think You Might Have an Eating Disorder

This is where it gets a little tricky.

Only you are able to admit to yourself if you need help beyond the RD. They will be able to give you guidance, and may have experience in eating disorders, but if you are struggling with the idea of gaining weight or increasing your caloric intake to where it is giving you serious anxiety, you probably need more than just a dietitian.

I have actually not been in this situation myself. I found it relatively easy to gain the weight. I was determined to do it, and therefore I could push out any nasty thoughts I had about what others would think of me.

That is not to say I did not look at myself in the mirror at times, seeing the extra weight on my body and feeling guilty about it, but I was able to reframe it and get on with my day.

There is a lot of history in my family with eating disorders, so I am very aware of it and have been around it most of my life. My mum had one until she was told by her doctors that she would never have children if she did not gain weight, which was enough to kick start her into recovery. It took her five years to fall pregnant, but here I am! I also have an aunt who has struggled with anorexia for 40 years and many friends who have had to work through it over the years.

Therefore, I know how much it can impact every moment of every day and how if it does not get treated early enough, it can be almost impossible to recover from.

I wish I had the right things to say or the words to help you overcome it, but I am just not qualified to do so. If you do suspect you might have an eating disorder, I would look for someone in your area who has worked with eating disorder clients in the past, and get some professional help. Again, the podcasts with Renee and Meg Steffey Schrier and Jessi Haggerty, along with Renee's book, *Orthorexia* might be a useful place to start.

Do I REALLY Have to Stop Running?

This is the question I get the most on almost a daily basis.

Is there any way to get your period back when you love running so much you just can't let it go?

Unless your body and mind was as beaten down as mine was after all those years, chances are you are reading this frustrated and fed up, but not quite ready to pull the trigger and stop running. Am I right?

Probably.

We have gone over the other options when it comes to gaining your period back. I would suggest trying all of the above before you head down this road, especially because just removing the running without doing any of the above might not result in your period returning… which would be soul destroying, as you have removed something you love and have nothing to show for it.

If you have tried everything else, and you are ready to go for it, or go "all in" as they say in _No Period. Now What?_, you are probably just reading this book for some moral support, in which case, you, my friend, are doing the right thing and I hope this book is helpful for you as you rest and let your body heal.

But if you are in the overwhelming majority who need that nudge, do you need to stop running?

The answer we all hate: it depends.

I have always been someone who decides on a goal, decides on something I want, and then I go get it. I will do whatever it takes to reach that goal and will make sure I do it to the best of my ability, so even though sometimes I may not get there, I know that I tried as hard as I could, so I have no regrets about the situation.

For me, with running, once I decided enough was enough, once I listened to my heart, which told me I wasn't in love with running at that point and I did want to start a family, I decided to jump through that window of opportunity, knowing full well that it could be fleeting AND if I didn't stop now, I could be damaging my relationship with running beyond repair.

So for me, it WAS a simple decision.

I was ready to step away and that did make it easy.

Don't get me wrong, it wasn't easy every day and I definitely had some inner turmoil going on as I went back and forth with my feelings, wondering if I was doing the right thing.

It was only when my friend Kat pulled me aside (a few days before I made the decision) and reminded me of something, something I will now remind you.

This ISN'T forever.

You could start this giving-up-running thing, get a month in and decide, *NOPE, this isn't for me. I want to go back to my old life of exercising 30 hours a week and being skinny.*

You always have that out.

Sure you will be a little out of shape and maybe have gained a few pounds, but your common sense will know that the fitness can come back pretty quickly and the weight will come off if you really want it to. This helps to set your mind in a place where it doesn't seem so scary.

However, I have a feeling you will be like me in that situation, and once you get that far, you will want to keep going, knowing that you have not come this far for nothing. The option is still there and always will be, but by then you will have decided you are stronger than that.

That is the thing about us runners, we are committed and we are determined. We want something, we go get it, and that is what you are doing.

Thankfully, we are in a sport where we can go back to running at ANY POINT. There are 5ks every weekend in almost every city, all you need to do is head out the door and you can run, and we already have the shoes…well, I am assuming you do!

As I have said in previous chapters, stopping running for a while is just the quickest way. If we want to think of it in running terms, imagine you went to live at altitude for your training, while everyone else was training at sea level (you stopped running while other amenorrhea warriors kept going, still trying to recover their cycles, but still running a little). You probably will get to your ultimate goal (overcoming amenorrhea) a lot faster with a little help from training at elevation (stopping running). It was tougher in the moment; training at altitude forced you to confront any doubt as your times slowed during the adjustment period (you had to really face those thoughts telling you that you are not enough and remind yourself that weight does not define you), but when it came to the time that mattered, race day, you were ready (you did the work, and your period came back).

I hope that analogy makes sense, it does in my head. ;)

I fell pregnant within three months of stopping running and I have heard from many other women who followed my path and had the same thing happen to them. If you do give up running, you are giving your body a better chance of success in less time.

BUT, as we already discussed, you can do it gradually if that feels safer to you. Backing off the mileage, slowing it down, cutting out the races, and just making running all about a little activity for health. It might take longer, but it can be done.

As much as my story might be a beacon of hope for many, that things can come together very fast, which helps in the early days of struggle, I also recognize that I was VERY lucky for it to come together that fast. For that reason, my story might become frustrating for you; maybe you will even end up resenting me. As much as the idea of that makes me sad, I also realize you have to do what is best for your heart and mental health.

For me to get my cycles back within three months of stopping AND fall pregnant on the first try, everything came together in a best-case scenario. We have to remember that everybody is different, and you may go all in, doing everything that you need to do, and have your patience tested for months on end, having that Bruce Almighty moment I mentioned to you earlier, yet still seeing nothing, no sign.

I am not going to lie, it will be frustrating as hell, and will make you consider whether it is even worth it. In much the same way that when we are in a race, we consider dropping out, wondering why we even bother, you will consider going back on your word, going back to your old life.

However, I know you have persevered through those rough moments in a race, making it to the finish line feeling even MORE proud of what you accomplished because you came so close to throwing in the towel. Well, here too, sticking with your amenorrhea recovery will also lead to an even greater feeling of pride the longer it takes.

It felt AMAZING when I resumed my cycle, and if you have to hang in there for longer than I did, every passing day will lead to it feeling EVEN BETTER.

It's not easy, but try not to compare your amenorrhea journey to others', especially mine. As the old proverb from Theodore Roosevelt says, "Comparison is the thief of joy."

I know, I know, easy to say, harder to do. I still find myself comparing to others, but unfollowing those people (yep, even me if it is painful) or hiding them, at least for the time being, can save your heart a lot of ache.

There is no wrong way to do this; you just have to decide which method is best for you. Maybe you even start with the slowly backing out method, changing a few things and then finding that doesn't work, but you are now ready to pull the trigger and stop running.

Or maybe making small changes is enough for your body to kick start the cycles again. You just have to decide how long you are prepared to wait.

I know you love running, but if you want a baby enough or care about your health enough, you WILL do what you need to do to get there. This may seem harsh, but at the end of the day, it is the truth. Anything worth having is worth fighting for, so you have to be prepared to give up something to get something really special.

I get it isn't fair that others don't have to go this far, but trust me, you will see that YOU actually hold the upper hand here; what you will learn from this process is a blessing, one you will be glad you went through.

Do I REALLY Have to Gain Weight?

I know, this is the part you really want to know and chances are, if you are reading this, you are a perfectionist who has always struggled with body image.

I am about to drop a bomb on you.

Ready?

I love listening to _The Power of Vulnerability_ by Brene Brown (would strongly recommend it), and she said this about perfectionism:

"Perfectionism is not the same thing as striving to be your best. Perfectionism is the belief that if we live perfect, look perfect, and act perfect, we can minimize or avoid the pain of blame, judgment, and shame. It's a shield. It's a twenty-ton shield that we lug around thinking it will protect us when, in fact, it's the thing that's really preventing us from flight."-Brene Brown

I think this very much applies in our situation, maybe we do want to look perfect, make everyone else think we are perfect, but the sooner we can accept that we are not perfect, nor will we ever be, the sooner we can get to being happy.

For now though, you are probably okay with the way you look (and would maybe even like to be a little thinner still). You want to overcome your amenorrhea and get your body functioning normally again, but the idea of gaining weight intentionally scares you half to death, especially as it has taken many years for you to reach a place you are happy(ish) with your body, nowhere close to perfect, but good enough.

I understand that.

When I decided it was time to address my amenorrhea head on, I was toned, fit, and lean…although I didn't really see it as much at the time. I thought I was still bigger than the other girls I raced against.

Now I can see that I was not.

I can see why other women would look at me with horror (or even disgust) when I would say that I was a bigger girl than other elites were.

Maybe when a well-wishing loved one commented to you about how skinny you were, you told them you were not THAT thin.

Here is a hard truth, my friend, one you probably won't like:

If you are in this position, and someone who loves you has made a comment about you being too thin, consider that you could be going through some body dysmorphia and you are actually a lot thinner than you think.

I know I was.

You might go to a mirror and look at the part of your body you don't like, the part you feel self-conscious about. Or maybe you see a photo of yourself and think about how huge another part of your body looks in that photo. That photo that was a moment in time. That photo that caught you at the wrong angle. Those photos that distort your reality and make you feel like you do need to slim down.

Don't believe that photo.

Rather than focusing on what does look good to you (let alone everyone else who thinks you look great!), you are criticizing yourself for the miniscule amount of imperfection you see.

If people close to you start making remarks, I know it can be easy to see that as a compliment, or if it is said in a negative way, that they are just being overprotective and maybe even jealous.

They are not. They care about you, and they want you to be healthy and happy. If those comments start coming through, you really need to listen. Especially if it is someone who means a lot to you.

What do they have to gain from telling you the truth?

They know you will probably be mad at them for saying it and it is a very awkward subject that most do not want to address, so if they have the confidence to say it, most likely there is a grain of truth in there, especially if you hear comments like that often, or if they are from someone who wouldn't usually make a remark like that.

About a year before I stopped running, during one of my trips in England, my dad hugged me and said with a tone of disappointment, *"Tina, I can feel the bones in your back."*

Part of me was proud. I knew that meant I was lean, fit, but the way he said it made me feel terrible.

The other part of me was in denial; it must have just been the way he was hugging me or maybe that he was just feeling insecure about himself; he had put on a few pounds over the previous years.

The comment stuck with me though, and I still remember it now because it was watering that seed of doubt that maybe I wasn't at a healthy weight anymore, maybe my body was struggling to keep up with what I wanted it to do.

My dad rarely makes any kind of comment about anyone else's appearance, and he has certainly never tried to interfere in my life, so that comment hit a nerve.

Has someone you loved made a comment like that recently?

If so, you might not like what I am about to say next.

If any of that above sounds familiar to you, I would say that yes, you DO need to gain weight, and it might need to be quite a lot. I know that is not what you want to hear, but you have to ask yourself, what is more important to you?

Would you rather look "skinny" in a bikini? Or have a healthy, happy body that is going to help you live many happy years?

Really, who cares how you look in a bikini? Honestly.

The people who see you on the beach either:
1. Love you for who you are no matter what size and shape you are.
2. They are people you are never going to see EVER again for the rest of your life.
3. They are looking at a photo of you after the trip to the beach, and they are feeling VERY jealous that you had such a fun time, and they are here sitting on Facebook.

And that's if they even notice your body!

How many people do you remember from years gone by at the beach/the-shopping mall/the grocery store? Or remember a specific photo of a friend and her size on her social media?

Not many I bet, and if you do, it is probably because they were doing something wacky or because they were doing something really unique that made you feel inspired (or they were making a really bad choice), not because they were a size 8 over a size 0.

At the end of the day, it comes down to this:

If you feel that you need to be a certain size, you need to be smaller to be happy, it is really not about the weight at all. It is what you have unintentionally focused on to control, as you feel a lack of control in another area of your life.

It is because you do not feel confident enough in who you are.

My friend, we need to help you see what everyone else around you sees. The chances are, you have lots of friends and family around you who love you and care about you very much. They see the beautiful soul that you are; they love who you are as a person, not what you look like.

I know that is easier said than done, and if we admit it to ourselves, it is not even usually about the ones who love us at all. We know they truly will love us as we are, but it is everyone else you worry about.

Trust me; I know.

We worry about the Facebook friends from years ago making the comment, *"Wow, she really let herself go."*

We worry about people we don't know who see our clothes that no longer fit, as our extra weight hangs over the top of our waistband as we bend down in Target.

We worry about everyone in the fitness world thinking that we are a lazy slob like the rest of the population.

I know; I felt the same way.

I loved knowing that people looked at me and thought I looked like I was in shape. As much as I would brush the comment off when people would make it about my arms being toned or my legs being *"to die for,"* I thrived on it. The idea of not having that anymore, or even someone making a remark about how I was now OUT OF SHAPE, was horrible to think of.

I wanted my body to work, but not that much.

But here's the thing, and you are not going to believe me when I say this, but **I feel more confident in my body now,** and especially after I got my period back, **than I did when I was at my leanest.**

I know you don't believe me, but it is true.

When I was at my peak, I would look in the mirror three, four, five times a day, tensing my abs, turning in the light, feeling frustrated that I never seemed to have a six-pack. I went through phases of stepping on the scale multiple times a day, in the morning and at night, allowing it to dictate my day. If it said I was "light" in the evening, I felt a thrill, a sense of accomplishment, and I would bounce out of the room, excited as I gave myself the permission to binge a little on candy in the evening.

If it said I was "heavy," my shoulders would round, my head would lower, and I would not allow myself to eat anything else that evening, no matter how hungry I was. I obviously had overdone it in the rest of the day, *body, you can wait until tomorrow.*

Until finally, one day I made Steve hide it, and that did, help get rid of those thoughts.

I would still find my eyes honing in on the negative every single time I saw myself in the mirror.

How was it different after I overcame amenorrhea?

I was at peace with my body; I was no longer fighting it. My body, so desperately wanting to get back to where it felt comfortable, safe, happy, and me desperately wanting it to reach this level of perfection that was impossible for it to achieve. Once I stopped fighting, I felt happy with who I was, not just the way I looked.

This adventure you are about to undergo is going to teach you so much about who you are, and although you might not believe me, you WILL come out the other side happier.

Think about it this way:

We all have our baggage, our insecurities, things that make us feel like we are not good enough. Those will continue to haunt you, appearing in various places around your life, until you address them, until you face them head on and deal with them.

If you overcome amenorrhea now, and learn to love who you are NOW, guess what? That means you don't have it hanging over your head anymore and you don't have to deal with it later...at a much worse time.

If you are taking the time to read this, you have an intention to overcome amenorrhea, which means your life must allow for you to at least try to work on it.

Especially if you are someone who is trying to get her cycle back to start a family, you want to make sure you work on this now.

Imagine if you have a little girl and someday you hear her talking about herself or even thinking about herself in the cruel way you think about yourself.

Makes you want to cry, right?

The same can go for little boys too; you still want him to grow up confident and feeling secure in who he is, and of course, to treat women with respect.

Most people who go through pregnancy worry about the weight gain, they are fearful of it and they come out the other side OBSESSING over the fact they need to lose the weight again. It makes them miserable and it makes it hard to even enjoy this new person who took nine months to grow into the beautiful little person they are, the person you gave your life to, and the person who brings you this level of love you didn't even know was possible.

How can you be the best mother you can be if you are obsessing over the way you look? That is taking your thoughts away from being grateful, thankful for this precious gift, and on to negativity and frustration.

If you stand up and face the voices telling you that your weight determines your happiness head on now, then when you are going through pregnancy and postpartum you will already have all the tools you need to accept your body for where it is, and you will give it grace that you are where you need to be.

Sure, I slip back into thinking about losing weight from time to time. I went through a few weeks of it around six weeks postpartum when I hadn't lost the weight I wanted to, but I was able to easily transition out of that by reminding myself of what I am telling you right now.

You are more than a number on a scale or a size of shirt. You are the beautiful, wonderful person you ARE.

A postpartum psychologist who will help you process all the other emotions going on also helps a little if you need extra support.

Would you rather deal with it now, while you have the mental capacity to do so, or when you are sleep deprived and overwhelmed with hormones after you have the baby?

I know what I would choose, and no, there is no way around it. Every woman will go through this at some point, especially those of us coming from a sport that has a focus on skinny=fast (although I think it is changing for the better!).

The choice is yours.

Ready to Take the Plunge and Stop Running?

Okay, so you have tried everything else, and you are finally at a point where this might be a reality. You have tried to wrap your brain around doing this, and although it terrifies you, you think you are ready.

If you are going to go "all in," going to take that time totally off and remove exercise, what are my recommendations for you to get through?

Find Penny

You already read the reasons why exercise can cause amenorrhea, so I won't go over that again, but you need to mostly keep in your mind that this time is all about reducing stress in your body, calming it down and letting it know that life is safe.

YOU are safe.

During this time, I called my period Penny, and I would imagine Penny as a little girl who had been in an abusive household. She didn't feel safe and was hiding in the corner of the room behind the couch. I would try to reassure Penny that she was okay and I would take care of her, but after all the years of abuse, she did not trust me.

Not really surprising though, right?

I had to take the time to get to know Penny (our inner little girl), show her that I did care for her, and I was going to give her a big warm hug as soon as she would let me. I was going to congratulate her for being so strong through these tough times by staying out of harm's way. For looking out for me, even though I wasn't there for her.

As she starts to feel a little more comfortable, Penny may poke her head out from around the corner, looking like she is curious, and start slowly edging her way out after you have taken a few weeks off or gained a few pounds (think of it as time you have spent just being in the room with her, showing her you are not going anywhere).

However, if you start exercising again, bringing intensity and stress back into the situation, or restricting your calories (think leaving, then bringing a ton of strangers into the room making noise or banging pots and pans and screaming), it will send Penny back cowering into the corner. You have to take the time to show her that you are not going anywhere. Both figuratively and literally, you are here to stay.

Imagining my period as a little girl made it a lot easier to deal with, because it then made it real. It made it easier to think about what I was doing and the decisions I was making, that they were having a real impact on another person. Even though she was imaginary, it helped.

I also liked the idea that it made it real in terms of I knew the end goal WAS a little girl...or boy, and I would NEVER want her to go through amenorrhea or the feelings associated with attaching our self-worth to the way we look. By working through this now and getting to a "normal person" weight, I would be limiting the likelihood that she would learn that the way she looked would determine who she was as a person.

If you want to take it one level further, you can imagine that Penny is friends with your future child. We know how much impact our friends can have on our own self-confidence.

This is where the journal came in.

Journaling

For me, this is one of the most powerful parts of the recovery process, especially if the end goal is to start a family, but you can also use journaling if you are doing this for health reasons.

I will explain the two scenarios you could be going through, depending on if pregnancy is the goal or if just overcoming amenorrhea for your own health is the goal. If you have never Journaled before, you will see just how powerful it can be. It will change the way you think about yourself, and make this seem much more manageable.

Now, I have to emphasize something first, and it is SO important to do this.

You HAVE to find yourself a meaningful journal.

Pleeeeassssee take some time finding one.

Find one with an inspiring quote, something about being on a journey or being brave, as that is what you are. Maybe it has a picture of a strong runner on the front, or a baby. Maybe it is about achieving your dreams and chasing down the impossible. You can also choose a plain one and decorate it yourself with stickers or images representing where you would like to be in five years.

As much as it is tempting to just use one you already have or just open a Google Doc or Word Doc, spend a little money on it.

Really. It will make it special to you, and it will make all the difference.

I would recommend a lined journal, but if you like writing freehand, by all means go ahead with the unruled.

Leave the first few pages blank; you may have something to add at a later date, maybe even a contents page if you are Ms. Organized and have the desire to at the end.

Now you are ready to begin the work.

Joy List

On the first working page, start a list of joy.

A list of alllll the things you enjoy (or think you would like to try), from the tiniest to the biggest.

This will be something you reflect on often, and start to work your way through during your recovery. Remember there is more to you than the way you look and the exercise you do, so really think about what things you enjoy doing. This is also a chance to have some fun with those activities or parts of your life you may have been neglecting in recent years for fear they might affect your training or your diet.

Your joy list should be full of things that bring a smile to your face, even thinking about them. It should be things where time just passes, you lose track of time, and feel like you could do them over and over. Some examples include:

- Meeting up with a best friend for a coffee.
- Eating cake batter ice cream in a waffle cone.
- Singing in the car to Backstreet Boys (oh, that one is just me then?).
- Getting a pedicure.

Use as many pages as you can, and of course, add to it as you think of new things…or even try new things you discover now you have all this extra time!

The Ultimate Bucket List

This is the next important step to prep yourself. This is your chance to go wild and really let your mind wander to the stories you would like to share as you sit in a rocking chair aged 85.

What would you like to do in your lifetime? What would you like to accomplish, have, see, experienced?

Make it as bold as you like, and make sure you take some time to think about this. You will definitely add things as time goes on. Don't forget to add the little trivial things that mean a lot to you.

Some examples from my bucket list:

- Represent my country in a world championship (CHECK!).
- Eat Chinese food out of a square box (you know, like they used to do in *Friends*! Don't ask me why, but most of my English friends want to do this at some point, ha-ha). For the record, I have NOT yet completed this one... I had Thai food in a box, but I am not allowing that to count, as my bucket list specifically says Chinese. :p
- Live by the beach.
- Raise beautiful, happy, healthy children (not yet checked, says childREN, not just child...besides, I don't know if she is happy yet. :p
- Go to Fiji.
- Run under 2:40 in the marathon (CHECK!).
- Meet Brene Brown.

You get the picture.

Be creative, be ambitious, and really give it some thought.

Gratitude List

The joy and bucket lists are one-off lists to be done at the beginning of your journal, and then you will continue to add to them.

The gratitude list should be completed every day, or every time you fill out your journal with your thoughts.

Turn to a fresh page and write the date in the corner of the page.

Now start to write all the things you are grateful for in this very moment.

All the things you are proud of yourself for. All the things you appreciate right in this moment. All the things that made you smile, even just a little, even if only for a second. They don't just have to be something that happened that day, but something that popped into your mind, maybe from the past that you were reminded of. Be sure to write it in first person.

The first time you do this will feel a little awkward, and maybe you don't feel like you have much to be grateful for on the surface, but they can be teeny tiny things to get yourself started. You will find it easier as you get used to doing it.

This will be things like:

- The man who held the door open for me today.
- That I have a good relationship with my mum.
- How good the cake was at the bakery this morning.
- When I won most improved in my freshman year of college.
- I am a kind person, who wrote a letter to Sally this morning.
- The funny cat video on Facebook that made me laugh.
- The beautiful blue sky outside.

Keep writing on every line (or as many as you can fit in) until the page is full. Take as long as you need.

Make sure you are not just going through the motions and writing:

- My mum loves me.
- My dad loves me.
- My brother loves me.

Really think about it.

No one is going to see this but you, so no one will be offended if they don't make the list for that day… In fact, maybe they should step it up

Once the page is full (go on to a second page if you like), take another read through. If you have done this right, it should put a FULL smile on your face, as you feel grateful for what you have.

Now that your journal is ready, let's go into a few scenarios and how to write in a journal for them.

If Becoming Pregnant is the Goal

Write to your future child.

Leave a few pages blank for things you might want to add before you give it to them, maybe words of wisdom or just a few quotes that mean a lot to you.

Make sure you write the date, and start to write to your future child as often as possible.

Write as if you are sending letters for them to read on their journey. Imagine they are on their way to you (no matter how far they have to travel). I used to imagine (what is now Bailey) on a train, excited to meet her parents, knowing she has quite a few stops along the way and a lot more to see and do before she arrives, but she is on her way.

One of my aunts often says that Bailey chose her parents well, and I love that way of thinking. It also reinforces the thinking that your future child is on their journey to you. It may take months, it may take years, but he or she knows who their parents are, and they are on their way.

Write in this journal any time you feel frustrated, sad, and angry.

Any time you see some skinny runner who gets her period every month.

Any time social media shows you pictures of someone running a PR and you wonder if those are a thing of the past for you (they are not; remember what I said Nancy said, maybe we can run faster with our bodies working how they should!).

Any time you feel lost or like it is never going to happen. It will bring you back to the moment, remind you of why you are doing this.

It is okay if sometimes it is a big negative, if it does turn into a venting session where you complain about life not being fair, that you really don't know if you are strong enough for this. Write it all out, get it out of your head and on to paper, and then imagine what you would tell your future son or daughter if they came up to you with the same problem many years later. What would you tell them? Write a response to them (yourself), and then read it back.

Of course, this has the bonus of helping you to start to visualizing that little person and what they are going to look like. This is an advantage of babies all looking pretty similar at birth; you can imagine whatever baby you like! In the end, it won't matter if they do or don't look like that. I was convinced Bailey was going to have dark hair like her daddy, so the little girl I imagined had dark hair, but now none of that matters… and I secretly love that she looks JUST like me as a baby, but shh, don't tell Steve. :P

You also might like to write to tell them about how the hotel is coming along.

In *No Period. Now What?* they talked about building a 5-star baby hotel, and this, above all else, was what I kept in my mind and took a few steps further. Gaining the weight and resting was nice fluffy, soft pillows and me building my baby a beautiful, state of the art hotel, complete with everything they needed. You would not want your baby staying in a crappy motel for nine months while they sleep on a futon with the bars digging into their back (think your bones if you are too thin). I would remind myself that the extra weight I was putting on was a fluffy pillow for her/him to put their head on and rest while they grew.

I like the idea of a hotel vs. a motel, because it really reinforces the idea that you are creating this body to be the best place it can be for your future child. It changes your perspective from taking something away to what you are GIVING someone else. Kind of the same thinking as when we do better as part of a team. You and your baby are going to be a team. The more you write about this, telling them what the hotel they are staying in is like, the more real it will feel.

If you like, you can also continue this into pregnancy, asking them what they think of the hotel you have created.

If Health is the Goal

This is almost the tougher one to do. Even though you don't have the pressure of wanting a baby sitting there on your shoulders, not having the "goal" at the end of this makes the motivation a little harder to define in those moments of doubt.

First off, you have to think about WHY you want to get your period back. You know in your heart (and your mind if you are reading this) that your body is not functioning as it should, and if you have had all the tests under the sun like I did, you will be feeling frustrated, because you ARE doing what you can, but it seems no one else cares (I do!!).

Journaling helps in this situation as it helps to remind you of who you ARE, not what you do.

Yes, you may be a runner (and yes, you still are a runner AND an athlete even if you are taking some time off right now). Even the best in the world have to take some time off sometimes, and they don't become non-runners during those times.

In 2017, Des Linden took a significant amount of time off running to get away from it, and then she came back in April 2018 to WIN the Boston marathon. If you listen to any interviews with her, she credits that time off as a critical part of why she ran so well at Boston.

For the record, I still consider myself an athlete and have the entire time; you should too!

You are a runner, but you are also a PERSON. A beautiful, wonderful, kind, loving, brave person. You wouldn't be taking this step if you weren't. You are thoughtful and sweet, you are funny and smart. You are everything you should be, and you need to remember that.

You can always go back to running. And remember, you can always start this, get a month in, and say, you know what; this doesn't matter to me, and go back to your old life. It is NOT forever.

BUT, I am pretty confident you won't do that, because I know you, you are dedicated, you are committed, and you are tough. You are going to see this as a challenge and you are kind enough to yourself as a person to take this step; you are going to beat this challenge, you are going to be the best amenorrhea recovery machine there could be.

After you have finished your joy list and bucket list for the journal, and have completed your gratitude list for the day, you are ready for the word vomit to come out.

Move to the other side of the page from your gratitude list, and begin to write. Whatever comes to your mind, DO NOT stop and think, just let the thoughts flow, and your writing should be pretty scruffy as the thoughts are flowing quicker than your hand can move. DO NOT edit (even if you make huge spelling errors or even miss words), just keep going, whatever comes to your mind.

I have found that for me, it ends up being frantic, like there are all these things tumbling out of my mind and I can't write fast enough. But you will get to a point where it all comes together and you start to see more clearly.

Your method may be different though.

Part of how you use this journal is going to depend on you as a person, how you like to journal, and how you are feeling. Once you have done this a few times, you will find it a lot easier.

I have given you the journaling PDF as a bonus with this book, containing specific instructions, that will help A LOT if you are stuck, but as someone recovering from amenorrhea, you might find it most helpful to start off writing in third person, as if you are giving yourself (or a friend, if that is easier to manage) a pep talk.

Mine would often start by writing to myself something like, *"Okay Tina, I know things are tough right now, you are being tested, and it does seem like the world won't give you a break, this is REALLY hard, but you are tough, you CAN do this!"*

Somewhere along the way, you should be able to switch over to first person, almost as if the person you are giving a pep talk to starts to respond, like in one of those motivational films where the underdog team suddenly "gets it," *"YEAH! I am tough! I am strong, you ARE right, I have been through worse than this, and I WILL get through this."*

Fill the page (and go on to the next if you would like) with this kind of talk. You should be writing out all those feelings of frustration, and then reminding yourself WHY you are doing this, WHAT you are doing to do it, and HOW you are going to do it. Write out all those fears and doubts and then respond to yourself.

This will be incredibly helpful for you to read in the future. Go back to it on tough days, to remind yourself how far you have already come and you will read little nuggets of wisdom you had from yourself on particularly good days.

During this time, I would recommend doing your gratitude list and journal every day, so you can document your journey, and read all those things you are grateful for other than being a runner or being skinny. You are so much more than that, and this will remind you of such.

Going from running being a part of your everyday life to not being there at all will be hard at times. I am not going to tell you it isn't. However, if you are determined to do this, you will be able to remind yourself that this is temporary and running will be waiting for you.

Other Recovery Secrets

If you are going to do the hard part, gaining weight and removing (or drastically reducing) your running, you do not want to go through all that to sabotage yourself in another way that really doesn't mean much to you.

In this next chapter, I will give you some additional things that will help you succeed in your recovery, and some suggestions for extra little things I did to assist with the return of my period.

Minimize Exercise

You want to make sure that if you are taking something you love away through stopping running or making it only short, easy miles, you are not going to stress out your body physically in another way.

There is no point giving up running if you are then going to walk 12 miles a day or go to Orange Theory, spinning, and CrossFit classes. The point of stopping (or reducing) your running is to calm your body down. Remember we talked about Penny earlier; you need to remind Penny that she is safe and that you are here to stay.

I know it can seem excessive, and make you feel like even more of a slob than you already do (even though it is not true!!), but the more you rest, like physically putting your feet up on the couch and instead of regular marathons, having Netflix marathons, the more safe your body will feel. The safer your body feels, the sooner it will bring your period back, especially when it is combined with additional calories.

Let's face it though, after years and years of exercise playing an important role in your life, maybe things do feel a bit empty. You will QUICKLY fill the time with other things (hopefully things from your joy list), but if you want to keep that sense of exercise for your own personal health of just getting outside in nature, by all means, go for a daily walk. Just make sure it is leisurely and short.

Call up a non-runner friend or walk with a family member (yes, especially those who do not walk that often; they will keep you humble and slow enough). Use the time to catch up, while getting out into fresh air. Or listen to your favorite podcast. I won't be offended if you do not want to listen to *Running for Real* at this time though!

Keep the walks to a max of 40 minutes, even less, if you can handle it.

I often fell into the trap of feeling like exercise wasn't "worth it" if it wasn't at least 45 minutes (or more accurately, an hour), but really, for this purpose, even a 10 minute walk once around your block is going to be good for you.

As for other classes, I had always wanted to do a trampoline class, and I did sign myself up while I still had amenorrhea. I gave myself 4 weeks of nothing, absolutely no exercise other than the odd, short walk just to be out in nature.

After that, I signed up for the class, but vowed this was for fun. This was not to prove I was the fittest trampoline-er or able to do more than anyone else, but just to have a bit of a laugh with a friend.

I am not going to lie, it was hard not to let my competitiveness take over and narrow my eyes to focus on being the best person there, but if you take a friend with you (who is not going to compete with you!), and then you can just laugh to one another.

It is okay to take some classes you have always wanted to try; be open to any class that has sounded interesting to you in the past, but limit it to one a week. Constantly remind yourself that pushing hard is only going to push your period away. If you can't hold back from the urge to compete, it is best to stop going.

Just make sure you give yourself a good 3-4 weeks of NOTHING before you start adding those in.

I also added in strength training after about a month; again, keeping the intensity down and doing it as if I was starting my strength training for the first time ever. You have probably built up to some pretty intense workouts, maybe even with heavy weights. Talk to your coach, or take your own program of what you feel is a beginner workout to a friend who has never strength trained before and either do it with them, accepting their feedback of whether it is too hard or advanced for them, or just share it with them, and see what they would think of it.

This is a great time to work on your mobility, your stretching, and foam rolling. Get your body moving in a way it never has before. Work out all those tight knots and restrictions that have been in there for years.

Especially if pregnancy is the goal, your body will thank you! If you can combine it with meditation, even better.

Remove Stress and Pressure

In many ways, this is actually the toughest one to do.

How can we remove stress? Especially if we are Type A planners?

It's pretty hard to just say *"I am gonna just chill, and be fine with a 6 hour Netflix marathon while I relax on the couch,"* but it is part of the recovery process, and it will only help.

You will be surprised how quickly you learn to embrace this part, even though at the start it might seem SO hard.

Once I started doing this, actually relaxing, I could feel the peace in my body. I allowed myself to believe that things will unfold the way they are supposed to. I believed that my journey would reveal itself, and I just had to trust.

The same goes for you.

Of course, I will always be a worrier, likely you will too, and as much as I or anyone else can tell you to not think so much, it's not as easy as that. All you can do is work on letting those thoughts go as much as you can. Think of your thoughts as clouds passing in a blue sky.

They are there, they may come over you, but then pass on.

Although it was scary to go through this process, and it brought a lot of highs and lows with my mood, once I got used to the new lifestyle, it was surprisingly enjoyable. I took comfort in knowing I was becoming a better person by facing those mental demons head on. You know, the ones who are probably in your ear too, telling you that you are going to end up unhealthily obese or that others will think you have "let yourself go."

Most people have to face these fears later in life, but I knew it was better to go through it before, learning to love my body and who I am. Meaning that I could enjoy pregnancy and the changing body because I already accepted that my body was more than just an appearance. It was mine to love and be proud of.

It wasn't easy, but I could tell very early on that it was going to be worth it. I just had to keep trusting and stay the course.

We fell pregnant on our first attempt, and I honestly believe a lot of it was because I just let off any pressure and expectation of it happening. Steve and I kind of had a *"well, we might as well try"* approach, rather than a "IT MUST HAPPEN NOW" approach, which we as driven people can easily end up thinking.

It was also the approach I tried to take when getting my period back. I have to admit, I was not ALWAYS successful with that mindset, it was hard not to think about it and want to control it, but I knew it would happen; I just had to be patient and give my body respect, give Penny respect.

When I chose to stop running and step away, I had not yet reached the point of resenting running (although I was close!), nor was I at the point that I was DESPERATE for a baby. I think that is yet another reason to start taking these steps early, cutting out the running early if a baby is the goal, because it may take a while. The way I saw it, the longer it took for me to get everything working again, the more likely I would be to channel all my drive and motivation into getting pregnant, viewing it as a goal I could complete by pushing harder, controlling more.

I knew deep down that getting pregnant doesn't work like that. You cannot FORCE it to happen. You can make it more likely, you can do little things that give you a higher chance (just as in running, we might take a supplement for the sake of improving a few seconds in a marathon), but at the end of the day, ultimately, we do not really have the final say.

The more you can take a relaxed attitude to resuming your cycles and getting pregnant, the better. Granted, I have already told you I was not the best at letting the cycles thing happen, so I get it, it's not easy. But if you can't let your mind rest as much as you would like, you can at least let your body rest by getting to know your couch, going to bed early, and becoming comfortable with being still.

Acupuncture

Another thing I started to do once I stopped running was going to acupuncture once a week or bi-weekly. I had heard wonderful things about acupuncture for fertility, but for me, it wasn't even really about the acupuncture itself and the effects it might have on hormones and fertility. For me, it was more about it was a time when I was made to relax. When you have needles sticking in your stomach and legs, you can't exactly move around. I vowed that I would use that time to truly rest, be still, and let my mind wander.

It helps to get you in the habit of being still, having nothing to do but let your mind wander.

Thankfully, my acupuncturist, Ramon, would leave me in there for up to 45 minutes once he put the needles in, and he would sometimes have me then flip over and have some on my back, leaving me another 30 minutes.

Acupuncture is expensive, so if I was going to spend my hard-earned money on it, I was going to make it worthwhile. This might be a good place for you to start too, because this way you can at least have that time once a week where you are in total rest...and you cannot physically move because if you do, the needles can hurt!

At first, it was tough to relax, and I am not kidding when I say sometimes I considered trying to reach for my phone or stash it under the sheet, but let yourself use the time effectively. You are putting your money into this; you don't want to throw it down the drain by not getting the full effect.

By putting in a monetary investment, it will make you stick to it, and for me, the acupuncture was well worth it, even if you remove the testimonials of thousands backing up the health benefits.

Yoga and Meditation

Another stress relieving option that could potentially do wonders for your recovery is going to regular yoga classes, gentle yoga classes mind you, not hot yoga or intense yoga.

At the more indie yoga studios, they will often have restorative yoga, which are classes that are veeerrrryyyyy chill and focus mostly around relaxing. Now, just a word of warning, you have to be in the right mindset for these ones. Sometimes if I was on one of those go-go-go days, I really struggled with them as they are all about holding a pose for 5 minutes and you will definitely NOT be bringing about any kind of sweat. BUT for your situation, while you are in recovery, they can do multiple things:

1. Force you to actually relax. This is yet another version of the acupuncture thing; you have paid for this class, driven yourself there, and so you might as well make the most of it, right?
2. If you can't shut your mind off as it is just racing…maybe this is exactly what you DO need… it probably was why I needed it so badly.
3. You will get some mobility work in, which kiiiiinda feels like exercise, without the sweat and stressing out your body part. You will leave the class feeling good about it, with an endorphin rush (okay, maybe a minute level compared to running, but it's something, right?).
4. Opportunity to meet other non-runner friends who don't know you as xx the runner. I met one of my good friends here in Lexington at a baby and me

yoga class, and she has no real understanding of what I do or what level of runner I actually was. I kinda like it that way.

If you do not have a restorative yoga opportunity near you, all yoga studios will offer a gentle or beginners' class. It might be a great place to trick yourself into thinking you are exercising, while really maximizing the relaxation and savasana part of class, which is what we need the most... even though I usually find it the most frustrating part!

I did not have it during this time, but I have since discovered *Headspace* and I strongly recommend it for bringing meditation in a different way. It is just 5-15 minutes a day, and the founder, Andy Puddicome, talks you through the entire thing, which is not so intense and easy to ignore. You kind of feel like you are doing him a disservice if you dared to cancel during. I wish I had this tool during my amenorrhea recovery time.

List of Joy

We have already talked about the list of joy and how to incorporate it into your journal, but now you need to start working your way through it.

This is fun, right?

You get to do those things that truly make you HAPPY.

I know you want to run, and you may feel that a lot of the joy in your life has been taken away from you. Not just the running itself, but all the things associated with it, like the sharing it to social media which leads to supportive messages from friends encouraging you, or the ability to meet up with runner friends. It may feel like without your running, what can you share? A picture of your cat? Your dinner? We all roll our eyes at those dinner pictures, *am I really ready to be one of those people too?*

But, let's think about it for a second; a lot of us end up missing out on SO MUCH because our running always takes precedence. Comes back to that idea of what are you GETTING instead of what is being taken away.

I have done that many times. Missing a friend's dinner at an Indian restaurant as I didn't want an upset stomach for my workout the next day, backing out on plans because I was just too tired from a long run, turning down ice cream as I really needed to eat healthy for my next race, and not even to mention all those cool classes and events we miss because we are out running and racing.

I loved being able to go to the farmers' market early on a Saturday morning or to check out what the city had to offer on a Sunday. When you remove running and step back, you actually open up a whole new world of excitement to make the most of, and it can be fun to work your way through your list of things to occupy your time.

Try some things you have ALWAYS wanted to do, and you never know what could come of it. Maybe you will discover a talent or a true passion for something you never had the time to pursue as your running took up so much of your time. Remember I told you about my friend Kat? When she stopped running, she was able to put herself into her music, which meant she gave it the time to see where it went.

And now? She is traveling the world doing gigs, writing albums, and making a career of her work! She would never have gotten there if she was still running seriously.

For me, that was not so much the case. I didn't discover a hidden talent for basket weaving or tightrope walking, but I did discover a lot of joy.

Being real with you, one regret though? Horse riding was on my list, but I never actually got a chance to do it (things happened too quickly!). That was not going to be a secret talent for me; I had already spent 10 years of my life riding horses as a child and teenager, but I did enjoy it.

It doesn't have to be something unique and exciting, it can be pretty simple things that just make you smile and feel good.

Some of the things I did during this time:
- Got peanut butter chocolate chip pancakes.
- Went trampolining.
- Spent time playing with my niece, Charlotte.
- Watched Ellen DeGeneres.
- Went for a walk early in the morning as the sun rose (I was always running!).
- Straightened my hair so it looked nice and dressed in nice clothes, so I felt confident.
- Played _Just Dance_.

The best one of all had to be meeting up with or calling people I had just not had time for before. I filled up a lot of my running time with communicating with my loved ones.

It really brought SO MUCH JOY and I could see they appreciated me being present with them, rather than squeezing them in when my running wasn't around, or thinking about how I had to get back because I had to be up early in the morning… or turning up with my hair in a messy bun, STARVING (and a little grumpy) because I had come directly from a run. Those wonderful, extended conversations ended up being so deep and meaningful, taking our relationship to a whole new level of closeness; it was amazing.

It might seem like you have had a lot removed from your life, like there is a void, but if you fill it with other people, even if that means doing something new and scary like volunteering, you will notice that not only does it fill that void, your joy and love for your life will soon be overflowing.

Our relationships really are the best things in our lives, above all else. YOU get the opportunity to have some amazing ones, especially with lots of extra time. You are driven and determined, which allows you to fit running in when others are too lazy; well, now you have some extra time that has appeared, and you can fill it with whatever you like, something that brings you joy in a whole new way. Not like running where you might enjoy parts of it but mostly enjoy the rush after no, pick the things where time passes by before you know it, you lose track of time as you are enjoying it so much. Those moments and the relationships, the memories that come with them, will give you a buzzing feeling that will equal, if not exceed, your runner's high.

Go Eat "Bad" Foods

I already mentioned this a little in the joy list, but I think it deserves its own section. Although it might be one of the scariest parts, especially when it comes to rewiring your brain, it is also one of the best bits and you can't even begin to imagine how jealous other people are going to be of you that you get to do this.

This is a once in a lifetime opportunity, and very few people actually get to have fun with this.

Go eat all those foods you have always wanted to eat. All the things on the menu that sound AMAZING, but almost immediately, that little voice says, *"Uhh no, that has too many calories/too bad for me/unhealthy/too much sugar."* For a little while, you have a free pass to GO CRAZY with those foods.

That is how I gained the weight I needed to get my cycles to resume in under 8 weeks. I cut the running out completely and ate whatever I wanted, whenever I wanted, primarily those "bad foods" I had ruled out in the past.

On the *Running for Real* podcast I had an episode with sports nutritionist Matt Fitzgerald, who has done a lot of research on what the best diet is for runners (and for people in general), and he talked about eating everything; yes, including fried food, sweets, and things people consider "bad."

If you are restricting a food group in any way, you might think it's "healthy," and it is, but that gets us in trouble. Same goes for my podcasts with Renee McGregor and Nancy Clark.

Unfortunately, as much as I hate to admit it (and maybe you won't believe me right now), this thinking of "bad" vs. "good" foods is what has gotten us into this mess in the first place; it is what meant that we didn't get enough calories to maintain our menstrual cycles. Maybe it wasn't that you cut those foods out; I know I didn't. I still had many of the foods I ate during this time, but the problem was, I would restrict after (or before) eating those foods to make sure I did not overload on calories that would then make me gain weight.

Whether you do what I did, and change the way you eat surrounding those foods, or you just don't even consume them at all, you have made food into a villain that is going to make you gain weight if you eat too much of it.

Now, this is the only time you are going to make that happen (gain weight), but not because you are eating those foods; those foods alone do not automatically make you gain weight, but once you are able to do this and you open the floodgates, telling your body that you are going to consume food, whatever food it wants and craves, as much as it needs, you will become hungry, VERY HUNGRY.

For the first week, I found that I was just eating for the sake of eating. I wasn't really hungry a lot of the time, but I was just making the most of the opportunity to eat extra, because why not? I figured every calorie extra from M&Ms or ice cream was helping me get one step closer to the weight that would get my cycle going again, why not do it with foods I loved the taste of, rather than foods that were calorie dense, but just okay.

After about a week though, I could not get enough. It was as if my body was saying, "For real? You are actually going to give me what I want? I don't have to ration food anymore? Oh my god this is the best thing eveeerrrr."

And boooyyy was I hungry, absolutely RAVENOUS.

I wanted to eat everything and anything in sight. I had barely finished one meal before I was hungry for the next, I couldn't get enough of sugar and sweets and salty and sour. I just loved it all.

I started to fear that I would never stop. My stomach would expand and get used to this volume of food and I would not be able to ever have control over my eating.

We hear about how addicting sugar and fats are, how would I ever be able to back off eating these foods all day long when I was enjoying them so much? I feared I would be so judged and everyone would look at me differently if I couldn't stop eating those unhealthy foods.

But I knew I had to trust the process, even if it meant that down the road, I had to do an intervention, put myself on some kind of diet to halt the hunger, but for now, I was gaining weight and I was feeling a lot better in every way.

The hunger continued for a few more weeks. I embraced it and just went for it. I remember going for a gastroenterologist appointment about the high AST and ALT scores in my blood work, and when she asked me about my medical state, I explained to her what was going on. When I told her I had gained almost 15lbs in 6 weeks, I saw her mouth open a little with shock.

I knew it was drastic; I also knew it was going to work. It wasn't long after this time that I started to notice changes in the way my body was acting, changes that were showing my periods were on their way. I was getting hot flashes, I was feeling full of energy, and my libido was back.

You can always gain the weight the "healthy way" by eating tons and tons of healthy foods, but really, are you then still keeping all those other foods in a category that you should always stay away from? It also makes it a LOT harder, because you have to consume such a big volume of those foods that you might struggle to get enough in, especially if you are still running.

If you had your favorite meal every single day for the rest of your life, eventually, no matter how much you loved it, you would become sick of it. That is kind of the approach here. If you let yourself go with whatever your heart desires, you are getting it out of your system.

One day I found I just woke up and I wasn't hungry anymore. The hunger was down to a normal person's hunger, and I found I could eat when I was hungry and stop when I was full. I didn't crave those foods anymore. I just wanted balance. I still enjoyed eating cookies and having a burger, but I also craved kale and beets.

This all happened once I reached the weight that I fell pregnant at. Once I reached the weight I last had my period at.

You might not believe me when I say this, as it was hard for me to accept when I was in the thick of it, but your body really will find equilibrium for you. Once you get to a weight where your body feels safe, it will stop craving those foods because it knows that it doesn't need you to eat those calorically dense foods anymore; you are safe.

Go Shopping

This will be one of the most terrifying parts, but also one of the best parts of this journey. Go get yourself a whole set of new clothes, or even a wardrobe full if you can afford it. I know, I know, clothes are expensive, and you love the ones you have, but they are going to destroy your confidence even having them around.

I did this after about seven weeks, when my body was starting to slow down with the hunger and I had a feeling things were starting to come together.

Using a Marie Kondo style method (she has a book called _The Life Changing Magic of Tidying_), gather up ALL of your clothes. Every single one of them. Get the ones from the closet downstairs, the ones hanging off the side of your couch, the ones on the floor of the backseat of your car, in your gym bag, and of course all the hanging ones and in drawers. Put them ALL in one place in one room.

Marie recommends holding each thing up individually and asking if it sparks joy in you. If it does, keep it; if it does not, get rid of it. However, I know from experience during this time that most of your clothes are going to bring you a level of frustration. Maybe they will bring joy in the future, but right now, right in this moment, all they do is make you want to cry because you cannot fit in them anymore.

I get it, and this part is hard, but I would try your best to go through them realistically to put them into two piles. One of clothes that you do love, you would still be wearing them often or you still do. The second of clothes that have run their course with you. Maybe that style has gone out of fashion, or maybe, like I found with many of my clothes, I never REALLY felt that good about them. It was one of those moments where you were in the store and it looked...uhhhh...okay, but you hoped when you got home you would feel confident and bold enough to wear it paired with some cute jeans (as opposed to the running tights and sports bra you were wearing when you tried it on, but it still never really made it out. Not enough to justify it staying.

Ask yourself, if your amenorrhea journey takes a few years, will you be interested in wearing this in two to three years' time when the fashion has changed? Did this ever really fit you in the first place?

Really be honest with yourself, even if that means the pile of clothes you are actually keeping is really small.

Once I had done this, I looked at the clothes I was keeping, and gathered up all the size XS (and many of my size S) clothes. I put them into a suitcase in another room of the house. I liked doing it that way as I was saying to myself, "it's not that I am NEVER going to wear you again, maybe I can find a way of being healthy and functioning while wearing you, but while I work on myself, you can go rest in a place where you do not bring me frustration." Take them out of the room, or at least out of sight.

From there, you might not be left with much. I think I had one pair of jeans and two pairs of shorts that fit me. I knew I had to go shopping.

Did I have the money to spend?

Not really, but I didn't just need clothes to feel better about myself, I also needed clothes to actually get on with my daily life. At this point, they were a NEED. My body physically could not fit into many of my past clothes...besides, for me, the goal was pregnancy, and I knew my hips would get wider for childbirth, so even if it wasn't about aesthetics, I would have to get some clothes that were bigger for that time anyway.

Go to your favorite store; get yourself a few outfits. Some things that are dressy for going out and celebrating your journey, eating those avoidance foods, and making memories, and then get some that are just casual and basic.

For me, I went to Express for my nicer things, for the things I knew should be of a higher quality and I wanted to take photos of myself in (hello, date night!). These are the things that will fit you and your body best; they are made better and therefore fit a woman's body better. I also went to H&M, another of my favorite stores, but let's be honest, the quality isn't amazing; however, it is cheap. I purchased a lot more from H&M, but that is because you can get a lot more for your money. I purchased a lot of plain semi fitted T-shirts in various colors, my everyday attire, and a few pairs of shorts, in slightly different sizes. That is one of the great things about these inexpensive shorts, you can experiment a little. I have about 6 pairs of shorts from H&M, ranging from 2-8, and they only cost around $10 each, so even if I barely wore them, I wasn't losing out on much.

Word of warning for H&M and many of the cheaper stores, their sizes vary WILDLY. Another reason I would recommend getting a few things from a nicer store, as I found H&M sizes came up TINY and many of them did not fit my body right. What you get is what you pay for, right? I could not believe I was purchasing a size I had never worn IN. MY. LIFE, and I am not gonna lie, it helped to fuel that thought of not being able to stop eating and ending up obese, but you HAVE to keep in mind that the labels in these stores are NOT accurate.

On that note, this is going to be tough to do.

Especially if you have been one size your whole life, and you see yourself going up one, two, three, four sizes. It is not easy, and I did struggle with it. But remember my friends; NO ONE can see that size but you! It is not as if we wear the size of our clothes on the outside, for the world to see. What is the point of squeezing into something that makes you feel "fat," destroying your confidence in the process, to say you are a specific number.

Firstly, that number does not define you IN ANY WAY. You are not a number, and this journey is hopefully showing you that. Not a number on a scale, not a number on a pair of jeans, not a number of years you have been struggling with this. You, yes YOU my friend, are the wonderful, beautiful, strong, courageous woman you ARE. And she is so much more than, so much better than, any one number. So yes, that might mean you go up a few sizes in your clothes, but your heart is also going up a few sizes as you are learning to give yourself and others compassion, love, and joy. Think of the Grinch and how his heart grew when he did good deeds. YOU are growing too, my friend.

You are also going to need some new workout clothes. It will be up to you whether you do this during your journey or if it will be too tempting to go out and use them. We all know how great it feels to go run or work out in some new running clothes, and if you feel the excitement is going to be gone if you purchase them and put them aside, if it feels like it is teasing, then save it as a reward for once you have your period back.

For me, I purchased a few things early on, and honestly, a lot of it was because I wanted to have some clothes that stretched, that were not so rigid in how they could fit, either requiring a belt as they were too big but I expected to soon fill them, or because they were too small but I didn't want to go and get something new yet. Running clothes are a little more forgiving, so if you get yourself some mediums, they will still fit you when you are smaller than that, but can also handle someone larger a little better.

I may have also kept many of my size small running tights out of the suitcase, as I could get away with wearing them for quite a while.

When to do this process?

You could sort your clothes and go get some new ones as a treat a few weeks into your journey and then use it as a form of reward for progress along the way, or you could just do it all in one go once you get your period back, as you reach your new normal. It will depend on your situation and how you are feeling.

If you are feeling a little down or sad, I would say that the money you will spend is WELL WORTH your mental health to go get yourself a few new things you feel good in. That will do wonders and help your recovery process.

And remember, have fun with this. How many other times in life do you get to go buy yourself a whole new set of clothes? I don't know about you, but I have never really done this before, and once I learned to ignore what the tag said and instead go for how I felt in it, I loved it!

Other Support

By now, you know of a certain book to read, I have only mentioned it 256 times so far. I would also take a read and then save this open letter I wrote for Self Magazine. This has my heart on a page, and I hope it speaks to you too, gives you words to encourage you along the way.

Join the *No Period. Now What?* support group on Facebook. The women in there are going through the exact same thing as you, and you will be amazed with the number of posts that are shared that feel like you could have written them word for word. Everyone is SO supportive, and it will help you to feel like you CAN do this, especially as many of the women stick around after (I am still in there!). It kind of helps you feel like part of a tribe, and you are all working towards the same goal, therefore so happy for one another as you reach the destination.

While I was on my leisurely walks, I would often listen to podcasts, and I found myself being frustrated with the lack of podcasts about either pregnancy or well-being that seemed to understand what I was going through.

They were all about being "healthy," as in trying to lose weight, eat more vegetables, and get rid of any fat you had on your body. They weren't just unhelpful, but in some cases, they were sabotaging. Making me question what I was doing, as this was the picture of health, right? Lots of fruits and vegetables and protein powder to get lean and fit. Here I was gaining fat intentionally and not exercising.

That is what gave me the idea for my Pregnancy and Postpartum Podcast Series I worked on while I was pregnant. I wanted to create a series of podcasts for women like me who wanted to fall pregnant in the near future. To know what to do when you are thinking about taking the leap to become pregnant, to answer ALL the questions you have once you are pregnant (and there are a LOT), and then how to get back into exercise again after having a baby.

I wanted to create something for us to listen to, to learn from, and to show us we are on the right track. Even though we might feel like salmon swimming upstream when everyone else is trying to lose weight, it would help us stay focused on the end goal: to start a family and get our bodies in a healthy place for us. Not for some celebrity or not for some skinny runner with skinny genes throughout her family.

While I worked on those podcast interviews, I did some interviews on my _Running for Real_ podcast about the topic. The first was bringing author of _No Period. Now What?_, Nicola Rinaldi, on the show. I decided to bring her on with Heidi Greenwood, who had been in a similar situation to myself, running as an elite, before deciding she wanted to start a family and stepping away from elite running.

I then did an episode with Tawnee Gibson once we both fell pregnant, to talk about the differences in our journeys. If you're not sure if you are ready for the all in approach, you can hear how Tawnee reached the same end goal without cutting exercise out at any point.

Finally, I decided I needed to address the issues and fears associated with food itself, especially for people like you and me to listen to when we heard those ads on the radio asking us if we need to lose 5lbs. Whenever those messages came on, I could listen to the words of these experts to remind me of not just why I was doing this, but why this is the right thing to do, even if the end goal isn't to have a baby.

You are doing this for your health. The episodes with Registered Dietitians Nancy Clark and Renee McGregor (author of *Orthorexia*) and the eating disorder special with Meg Schrier Steffey and Jessi Haggerty are absolute gold, and you can find them for free any time you like. Anytime you need reminding that you are doing this for the best of your body, and that it is okay to eat all foods, even the ones you have always feared.

Some other non-running podcasts I would recommend checking out during this time:

Life Unrestricted with Meret Boxler - this one is made for us!
Happier with Gretchen Rubin
Mind Body Musings with Maddy Moon
Real Health Radio with Chris Sandeli
RD Real Talk with Heather Caplan
The BodyLove Project with Jessi Haggerty

Each of these not only has at least one episode covering amenorrhea, but they focus on body positivity and feeling more confident in who you are and the difficult decisions we make, something that is needed at this time.

I would also once again recommend my pregnancy and postpartum podcast series if you are trying to get pregnant.

So what next?

Well, the next part of your journey is up to you, my friend. I have given you advice on every single area I have worked on to get my body functioning again and I have shared advice from some of the experts I have learned from during my recovery process.

Now what is left to do is DO IT.

I know, that is the one thing you don't want to do.

Can't I just keep reading about it, maybe more reading will give me more reasons to do it, and then I will finally be motivated to go for it?

I am afraid not. I have covered over 100 pages, and that is more than enough to get you going.

It is scary, I am not gonna lie, you are going to feel like you have it all wrong while everyone else around you is talking about losing weight. Whenever anyone starts to talk about their body in a negative way, to lose weight or not, I would strongly suggest removing yourself from that situation. You do not need their insecurities too, we have enough of our own! Go listen to one of those podcasts I mentioned to counter that!

It is going to be hard, it is going to force you to face whatever demons and insecurities you have, but it WILL be worth it.

Go do it, you ARE strong enough.

Originally, I was going to save this section for those who had resumed their cycles, as kind of a "well done" for your hard work, but after talking to Dr. Rinaldi about it, this would also be helpful for you if you are still in the thick of it, especially if you are struggling with your visualization practice.

If you have got your period back, and have saved this section for that, these words will speak to your heart in a very powerful way, but if you are reading it while still working, they might provide an insight into just how good it is going to feel when it comes together and you get that sign that it is here.

The choice is yours. :)

YES! I Have My Period Back!

It just happened!

The moment you have thought of for all those hours, envisioned it happening, and here it is! You looked down in your underwear and saw it! You know your body is back on track, and you have done the work to get it there.

Although I didn't get the blood in my underwear as I fell pregnant before I got the chance, I did find out I was ovulating, and I remember the absolute HIGH it brought me, as good as any race celebration.

It is kind of like that, right?

You have been training for MONTHS or even years for this, and you have finally achieved it, the one goal you had. It wasn't easy, you went through many struggles, moments of doubt, moments where you considered quitting and wondered what the hell you were doing this for, anyway. But it is here!

And booooyyyy is it worth it!

Well done, my friend. YOU have put in the work, and now you have the reward to show for it.

Does your body look THAT different? Probably not. I am sure you have been receiving some compliments from loved ones about how great you look. They are not just doing it for the sake of it, as they know how hard you worked (although yes, there will be a little of that), but they do actually mean it.

At first, I thought my loved ones were just saying it because they knew I was feeling a little unsure, but after a while, I started to ask some of them if they really meant it, or if they were just saying it for the sake of saying it.

EVERY SINGLE ONE said they promised they meant it. That I looked healthy and happy, glowing almost, because my body was no longer grey from the hard training that was tearing me down day after day. They couldn't feel the bones in my back as they gave me a hug anymore. They had the Tina they loved back again, the one who genuinely listened to what they were saying and didn't seem to be distracted or too exhausted to really pay attention. They meant every word, and I bet your loved ones do too. To this day, I am still getting compliments, and now my friends and family tell me that I look so much better than I did as an elite.

And what about you?

Do you feel more confident?

I know I did. I could barely believe it, but somewhere along the way, I stopped caring about my belly in the mirror. I stopped caring or even wondering if people would think I was "getting fat," I stopped thinking about the number on the scale. It just doesn't matter anymore.

For me, knowing having a baby was eventually the goal, I still kept in my mind that I was building a nice, soft, fluffy pillow for my baby to sleep on. I was going to build him or her a Hilton hotel on the oceanfront, with a lovely soft bed, complete with squishy pillows, not a Motel 6 with bars in the bed you can feel as you sleep. That made it easier to go beyond the numbers, but I did start to notice that just in general I felt better. Mostly after the shopping, getting clothes that actually fit me, and once I realized that no one actually knew I was wearing a size six instead of a size 2 (size 10-12 in UK vs. 8).

I finally had some decent boobs, too. I could wear one of those tops with a plunging neckline that cuts down the middle with or without a bra! The ones I had always seen women wear, but figured it looked silly on someone with very little chest. Having boobs I could actually be proud of helped a lot.

I also noticed my body just felt more feminine. I can't put my finger on what it was, but I had always...okay, not always, but since I had amenorrhea, had a kind of boy-ish shape to my body. Some small curves, but overall, mostly straight up and down. I loved that I now had a womanly figure. Not quite hourglass, as I had also added weight around my waist, but it just felt good.

I felt good. In energy levels. In who I was. In what I looked like.

I finally came to the realization that skinnier was not better. I had come a long way, and likely you have too if you are reaching this point. It feels good, doesn't it?

I am not saying all the time, of course a small part of you will always want to have that lean body, look like the models we see in magazines, minus the perfect skin (airbrushed of course), legs that go on forever (nothing we can do to change that!), and abs of steel (when they also haven't eaten anything in a week). It is only natural to want to be back there when we are told that is beautiful.

However, I am hoping you have also found that YOU are beautiful.

YOU.

Not your body. Not your hair or your face. But YOU, the person inside.

I bet your family and friends are SO excited to have the person they know and love back. The one who doesn't get all nervous and jumpy when they suggest going to that new burger restaurant or going out to get appetizers before a night out. They love you for you, and now that you have your period, and hopefully your confidence back, guess what?

You get to go ENJOY this life!

You can start adding running back in (although I would probably recommend giving it a few more months before you do that, maybe add in some strength training or light fitness classes once or twice a week first), but you also have discovered that you have a whole life, a whole host of things that bring you joy that you can now keep in your life.

Although I did start running as soon as I found out I was pregnant, that was only because I knew that at that point, I really couldn't do myself any harm when it came to my body functioning. If I was pregnant, I was already on this nine month course that was just going to go along regardless of whether I ran or not.

I kept it VERY easy and VERY short because of paranoia of a miscarriage (although again, my pregnancy and postpartum series will explain all about running in pregnancy), but had I not fallen pregnant that fast, I probably would have kept off the running for another few months until I knew my body had totally regulated. That is what I would suggest for you.

My first menstrual bleeding in 10 years started on December 24th, 2018, 11 months after I gave birth to Bailey. As you know (or will soon know), it is the most incredible feeling, one that only we can understand. To know that your body is functioning, happy, and healthy. That you did the work, and you are now receiving the reward.

Some women will get theirs back a lot sooner than 11 months, but others do not get theirs back for up to three months after they stop breastfeeding completely. If you are postpartum, there will be many other variables that come into this. However, you must keep in mind that your body is sensitive to calorie deficits; you would not have had amenorrhea in the first place had that not been the case. The best advice I can give to you is to eat, more than you think you need, and if you are unsure, eat more. It is far better to be overfueled than underfueled.

If I am even remotely hungry, I eat, because I know I am burning off a lot running and breastfeeding...let alone the calories burned looking after the baby! I found my body settled around a certain size, and as it seems to have stayed there, this is my happy weight, where my body wants to be. Probably 10-15lbs higher than it was while I was at my peak as an elite, but that doesn't matter; it is fueled and happy there.

I hope getting mine back while running 70 miles a week has proved I do not have to cut out the running again when we want to try for another child. I hope that eating enough, noticing my body has settled, and of course, my period returning, mean that I will not end up in RED-S again. I imagine this is where my body wants to be, especially without overthinking food.

I am not claiming to know all the answers or that I have overcome it forever. I am not above you or anyone else. This book is about what I did to get my body to a healthy place, which has hopefully provided you with comfort and camaraderie. This book is for me to support you on your journey, but in the future, who knows, you may be the one supporting me if I end up back down the amenorrhea path again someday.

For now, though:

You have earned the right to celebrate, so go do it.

Just a word for friends who get their cycles back, but are struggling to get pregnant:

I can't give you any advice on this, nor would you want me to. Especially as someone like me who fell pregnant on the first try probably makes you angry. Anything I would say could come out incredibly patronizing and frustrate you further.

One thing I will say though, a friend once told me that if you are unsuccessful, you should go out for sushi and wine with your partner, or beers with medium rare burgers with blue cheese. Eat the foods and drink the things you will not be able to when you are pregnant. Celebrate the love you share with your partner and go enjoy those things.

Heck, enjoy being able to go out together at all. I can count on one hand the number of dates Steve and I have had since Bailey was born; it isn't many. Enjoy being able to wait an hour to eat at a very popular restaurant (if that happened now, we would turn around and walk out the door), enjoy going to fancy restaurants where you can get dressed up and have a five course meal over two hours. Go to the cinema, a crude comedy club, a concert.

Do all the things you will no longer be able to do once you are pregnant or have a baby. I wish I had done more of those during that time.

Keep on having fun with this new lease of life!

My Final Words to You, My Friend

Well, this book ended up being a heck of a lot longer than I ever expected. Maybe I did have more to say than I thought. My goal with this book was to give you everything I know about amenorrhea.

Sure, I could have paid more attention to the sciencey stuff along the way, learning why this was happening. It could have made things easier to explain to loved ones who were asking about it, or even explaining it to you.

But for me, I am just not all about that. I wanted to get to the end goal, and just as I am not interested in the details of training, why mile repeats should be done on the 5th week and 11th week of your marathon plan because they...well, I don't even know, but this is what Steve is ALL about (find his training plans here).

For me, it doesn't really matter so much WHY this is happening; I just wanted to fix it.

If you do want to find out more about the why, understand the science behind what is going on beyond what I have shared from the experts in this book, there is a whole lot of research coming out now and you will find plenty.

I hope this book has shown you that I understand. I get how scary it may be, and I know you are going through a lot. I hope it helps just having someone who gets it, especially when the rest of the world might wonder why you are acting all strange and have suddenly stopped running.

A family friend recently told me that she had no idea why I got so much attention when not every runner had a period. Why was I seen as some kind of role model? It was a known thing that runners didn't get their period, she told me.

Wrong. And ouch!

There are plenty of us, but it is certainly not everyone!

I might not be able to send many words of encouragement to you individually, but I hope this book will show you that you are not alone, that you CAN fix this, and, my friend, you will.

One more hard truth to finish:

Only YOU can do this. You have to want it enough. You can go to all the therapists, endocrinologists, dietitians, acupuncturists in the world, but they aren't going to be able to help you AT ALL, if deep down, you don't want to be helped.

If you really do want a baby, go build that 5-star baby hotel.

If you want your health back, go get it.

This is YOUR life, no one cares as much as you do, and the old saying is true, others will only learn to truly love you when you learn to love yourself first.

You are a beautiful, wonderful person, regardless of what you look like. I hope you will allow yourself to see that. Talk to yourself the way you will talk to your daughter or son. Give yourself kindness and grace. Understand that it will take time, hard work, and energy.

But you know from being a runner or a fitness lover that nothing worth having comes easy. The longer the journey takes, the further outside of your comfort zone you have to go, the better it feels at the finish line.

Your finish line is regular cycles, and you ARE going to get there. You just have to decide if you are going to put your head down and show up now, or if you are going to wait a few years to achieve that goal.

You can do it. I know you can.

Now go make that happen.

Hi, friend!

Will you do me a HUGE favor?

If you found *Overcoming Amenorrhea* to be helpful, would you mind taking a moment to write a review on Amazon (or on my website, if you purchased it there), please? Even a short review helps, and it means a lot to me.

If someone you know is struggling with amenorrhea, or if you even suspect that maybe she is, with all her injuries or setbacks, please send her a copy of this book.

If you could gift it to her through Amazon, you will help us both!

THANK YOU!

Finally, if you would like free bonus materials that I guarantee will help you to feel better about who you are (adapted from the work of a famous psychologist), and see that you have so much more to offer than just being a runner, go to tinamuir.com/oa-bonus

You can find me on Instagram @tinamuir88, Twitter @tinamuir, Facebook.com/RealTinaMuir, and don't forget to come join the Running for Real Superstars community on Facebook at tinamuir.com/superstars.

You are a wonderful, beautiful person; I believe it, go see it for yourself!

Resources

De Souza MJ, et al. "Luteal Phase Deficiency in Recreational Runners: Evidence for a Hypometabolic State." *Journal of Clinical Endocrinology & Metabolism.* 88(1) 2003: 337-46.
https://academic.oup.com/jcem/article-lookup/doi/10.1210/jc.2002-020958;

De Souza MJ, et al. "High Prevalence of Subtle and Severe Menstrual Disturbances in Exercising Women: Confirmation Using Daily Hormone Measures." *Human Reproduction.* 25(2) 2010: 491-503.
https://academic.oup.com/humrep/article-lookup/doi/10.1093/humrep/dep411

Hill EE, et al. "Exercise and Circulating Cortisol Levels: The Intensity Threshold Effect." *Journal of Endocrinological Investigation.* 31(7) 2008: 587-91.
http://link.springer.com/article/10.1007%2FBF03345606

Mastorakos G, et al. "Exercise and the Stress System." *Hormones.* 4(2) 2005: 73-89.
http://www.hormones.gr/57/article/article.html

Berga SL, Naftolin F. "Neuroendocrine Control of Ovulation." *Gynecological Endocrinology.* 28(Suppl 1) 2012: 9-13.

http://www.tandfonline.com/doi/full/10.3109/09513590.2012.651929

Stubbs RJ, et al. "Rate and Extent of Compensatory Changes in Energy Intake and Expenditure in Response to Altered Exercise and Diet Composition in Humans." AJP: Regulatory, Integrative and Comparative Physiology. 286(2) 2004: 350R-58. doi: 10.1152/ajpregu.00196.2003

Mountjoy, 2014.
https://bjsm.bmj.com/content/bjsports/48/7/491.full.pdf

Podcasts Mentioned

Pregnancy and Postpartum Series

Running For Real Podcast with Nicola Rinaldi and Heidi Greenwood

Running For Real Podcast with Tawnee Gibson

Running For Real Podcast with Nancy Clark

Running For Real Podcast with Renee McGregor

Running For Real Podcast with Meg Steffey-Schrier and Jessi Haggerty

Running For Real Podcast with Matt Fitzgerald

Running For Real Podcast with Bhrett McCabe

Running For Real Podcast with Trent Stellingwerff

Running For Real Podcast with Guy Winch

Life Unrestricted Podcast with Meret Boxler

Happier Podcast with Gretchen Rubin

Mind Body Musings Podcast with Maddy Moon

Real Health Radio Podcast with Chris Sandeli

RD Real Talk Podcast with Heather Caplan

The BodyLove Project Podcast with Jessi Haggerty

The Power of Vulnerability by Brene Brown

Books Mentioned

No Period. Now What? By Nicola Rinaldi

The Life Changing Magic of Tidying By Marie Kondo

Orthorexia by Renee McGregor

Other Suggested Services

Inside Tracker

Nourish Balance Thrive.

Running For Real Training Plans

Headspace

Sports and Cardiovascular Nutrition Dietary Practice Group of the Academy of Nutrition and Dietetics

Running For Real Superstars Community

Other Reading Materials

FREE bonus materials for you about feeling good in who you ARE

Letter to runners with amenorrhea in SELF Magazine

Runners World article

People Magazine article

Blog post on stopping running

Train Brave Campaign

About the Author

International elite runner for Great Britain and Northern Ireland, Tina Muir is a mother and former professional runner (and maybe one again someday!) who shocked the running world by stepping away from the sport at the peak of her career to overcome her amenorrhea of nine years. Having run a personal best time of 2:36 in the marathon just three months before, Tina brought awareness to the issue of amenorrhea, the cessation of menstruation, by sharing her story. Dozens of outlets covered Tina's story, including *People* magazine, *Outside*, *Runner's World*, ESPN, *Women's Health*, *Glamour*, and many more.

Tina was voted one of the 21 women changing the running world for the better by *Women's Running* magazine in 2017, and in 2018, she became the first cover model of a fitness magazine to be featured with a running stroller (and her daughter, Bailey) for the October issue of *Women's Running UK*. Tina has written articles for the *Guardian*, *Runner's World*, *SELF*, and *Mind Body Green*.

Tina is the founder of Running For Real, a community, podcast, and website for runners to share their true selves and grow to become better people. The *Running For Real podcast* has amassed over 1.1 million downloads in the first 18 months of release, and regularly features in the iTunes best Health podcasts chart.

Tina lives in Lexington, Kentucky with her daughter and her husband, Steve.

Printed in Great Britain
by Amazon